GoodFood
Low-calorie recipes

10 9 8 7

Published in 2013 by BBC Books, an imprint of Ebury Publishing
A Random House Group company

Photographs © BBC Worldwide 2013
Recipes © BBC Worldwide 2013
Book design © Woodlands Books Ltd 2013
All recipes contained in this book first appeared in BBC *Good Food* magazine.

The Random House Group Limited
Reg. No. 954009

Addresses for companies within the Random House Group can be found at www.randomhouse.co.uk

A CIP catalogue record for this book is available from the British Library

Penguin Random House is committed to a sustainable future for our business, our readers and our planet.
This book is made from Forest Stewardship Council® certified paper.

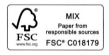

MIX
Paper from
responsible sources
FSC® C018179
www.fsc.org

To buy books by your favourite authors and register for offers visit www.randomhouse.co.uk

Printed and bound by Firmengruppe APPL, aprinta druck, Wemding, Germany
Colour origination by Dot Gradations Ltd, UK

Commissioning Editor: Muna Reyal
Project Editor: Joe Cottington
Designer: Kathryn Gammon
Production: Beccy Jones
Picture Researcher: Gabby Harrington
ISBN: 9781849906852

Picture credits

BBC *Good Food* magazine and BBC Books would like to thank the following people for providing photos. While every effort has
been made to trace and acknowledge all photographers, we should like to apologise should there be any errors or omissions.

Will Heap p43, p47, p63, p83, p107, p109, p113, p131, p163, p209; Lara Holmes p167; Jonathan Kennedy p93, p97, p127, p133, p161;
Adrian Lawrence p85, p139; Gareth Morgans p23, p75, p105, p129, p183; David Munns p19, p25, p29, p31, p33, p35, p51, p59, p71,
p79, p87, p91, p101, p119, p135, p137, p141, p151, p154, p157, p175, p177, p185, p187, p193, p197, p207, p211; Myles New p15, p27,
p37, p39, p65, p67, p69, p89, p121, p149; Stuart Ovenden p21, p45, p49, p61, p73, p111, p173, p179, p181, p195; Lis Parsons p11, p17,
p41, p55, p77, p81, p95, p123, p145, p147, p153, p159, p165, p169, p171, p191, p199, p205; Howard Shooter p99, p117, p125; Maja
Smend p13, p53, p201, p203; Simon Smith p189; Yuki Sugiura p115; Isobel Wield p57; Jon Whitaker p103, p143.

All the recipes in this book were created by the editorial team at *Good Food* and by regular contributors to BBC magazines.

healthy

GoodFood
Low-calorie recipes

Editor **Sarah Cook**

BBC
BOOKS

Contents

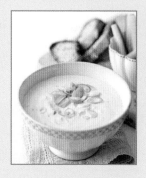
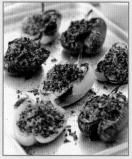
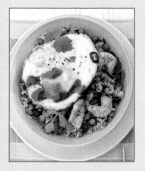

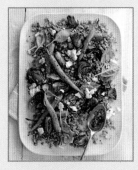 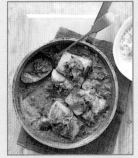 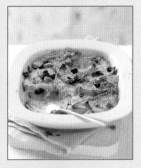

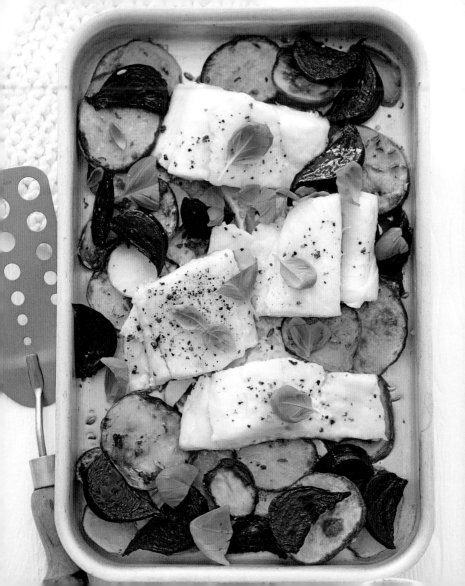

Introduction

After trying every crazy diet out there, we've gone back to basics and realised the easiest and most sensible way to lose weight successfully is simply by counting the calories – so we are! And we've created this fantastic little book so you can join us, too.

Throw out your calculator. Who wants to waste time struggling with complicated maths when we've done all the hard work for you? Every single recipe has a calorie stamp, telling you clearly and accurately how much is in every portion – and if that weren't clever enough, we've even divided the chapters into calorie ranges, so it literally only takes a second to find something to suit you.

We've delicious ideas for breakfasts, lunches, snacks and suppers, so you can throw out every other diet book cluttering up your shelves – we've got it all covered. And there is even a special chapter full of yummy cakes, bakes and puddings so you can keep eating healthily but still enjoy those treats you love so much, including an absolutely scrumptious Lighter Chocolate Tart.

Think you have to give up curry? Think again. How does a tasty Low-fat Chicken Balti sound? Or worrying that you will lose your willpower and reach for the takeaway menu? There is just no need when we've got a recipe for Thai Fried Rice with Prawns & Peas for less than 300 calories per serving – wow! And if you are trying to balance a healthier lifestyle with feeding your family, then we've got plenty of tasty recipes that you'll come to rely on, like our Beef & Bacon Meatloaf, Cheesy Bean & Sweetcorn Cakes and Easy Chicken Pies.

In fact, when you are cooking from this little book, you might forget you're on a diet altogether! So what are you waiting for? Pick up a copy and prepare to enjoy the easiest and tastiest way to shape up that you have ever tried.

Sarah

Sarah

Notes and conversion tables

NOTE ON CALORIES: If a serving suggestion is not listed in the ingredients or mentioned in the recipe title, it has not been included in the total calorie count. If you choose to follow the serving suggestion, you will consume additional calories to the number stated in the recipe.

OVEN TEMPERATURES

Gas	°C	°C Fan	°F	Oven temp.
¼	110	90	225	Very cool
½	120	100	250	Very cool
1	140	120	275	Cool or slow
2	150	130	300	Cool or slow
3	160	140	325	Warm
4	180	160	350	Moderate
5	190	170	375	Moderately hot
6	200	180	400	Fairly hot
7	220	200	425	Hot
8	230	210	450	Very hot
9	240	220	475	Very hot

APPROXIMATE WEIGHT CONVERSIONS
• All the recipes in this book list both imperial and metric measurements. Conversions are approximate and have been rounded up or down. Follow one set of measurements only; do not mix the two.
• Cup measurements, which are used by cooks in Australia and America, have not been listed here as they vary from ingredient to ingredient. Kitchen scales should be used to measure dry/solid ingredients.

NOTES ON THE RECIPES
• Eggs are large in the UK and Australia and extra large in America unless stated otherwise.
• Wash fresh produce before preparation.
• Recipes contain nutritional analyses for 'sugar', which means the total sugar content including all natural sugars in the ingredients, unless otherwise stated.

SPOON MEASURES

Spoon measurements are level unless otherwise specified.

- 1 teaspoon (tsp) = 5ml
- 1 tablespoon (tbsp) = 15ml
- 1 Australian tablespoon = 20ml (cooks in Australia should measure 3 teaspoons where 1 tablespoon is specified in a recipe)

APPROXIMATE LIQUID CONVERSIONS

metric	imperial	AUS	US
50ml	2fl oz	¼ cup	¼ cup
125ml	4fl oz	½ cup	½ cup
175ml	6fl oz	¾ cup	¾ cup
225ml	8fl oz	1 cup	1 cup
300ml	10fl oz/½ pint	½ pint	1¼ cups
450ml	16fl oz	2 cups	2 cups/1 pint
600ml	20fl oz/1 pint	1 pint	2½ cups
1 litre	35fl oz/1¾ pints	1¾ pints	1 quart

Good Food are concerned about sustainable sourcing and animal welfare so where possible we use organic ingredients, humanely reared meats, sustainably caught fish, free-range chickens and eggs and unrefined sugar.

Courgette & tomato soup

Make this soup in late summer or early autumn, when courgettes and tomatoes are plentiful and cheap. It freezes well, so a big batch will keep you going through winter.

90 KCALS

TAKES 45 MINUTES ● **SERVES 8**

1 tbsp butter

2 onions, chopped

1kg/2lb 4oz courgettes, sliced

1kg/2lb 4oz tomatoes, chopped

2 tbsp plain flour

½ tsp turmeric powder

2 litres/3½ pints chicken or vegetable
stock from cubes

1 Melt the butter in a large pan, add the onions and courgettes, and cook for 5 minutes on a medium heat, stirring occasionally.

2 Add the tomatoes and flour. Cook for a couple of minutes, stirring around to stop the flour from becoming lumpy. Add the turmeric and stock, then cover and simmer for 30 minutes.

3 Purée in a blender, or with a stick blender, then push it through a sieve if you want a really smooth texture. Serve, or chill and then freeze for up to 2 months.

PER SERVING 90 kcals, protein 4g, carbs 12g, fat 3g, sat fat 1g, fibre 4g, sugar 8g, salt 0.8g

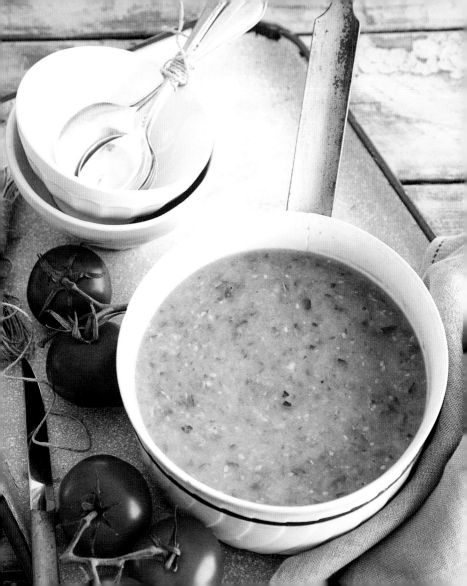

Beetroot houmous

If you love houmous, try this healthy version – it's much lower in fat than the ready-made stuff, and the beetroots add a lovely sweet note.

90 KCALS

TAKES 1 HOUR, PLUS COOLING
- **SERVES 8**

500g/1lb 2oz raw beetroot, leaves trimmed to 2.5cm/1in, but root left whole

2 x 400g cans chickpeas, drained and rinsed

juice of 2 lemons

1 tbsp ground cumin

natural yogurt, toasted cumin seeds and a few torn mint leaves, to garnish

1 Cook the beetroot in a large pan of boiling water with the lid on for 30–40 minutes until tender. When they're done, a skewer or knife should go all the way in easily. Drain, then set aside to cool.

2 Pop on a pair of rubber gloves. Pull off and discard the roots, leaves/stalk and peel of the cooled beetroot. Roughly chop the flesh. Whizz the beetroot, chickpeas, lemon juice, cumin, 2 teaspoons salt and some freshly ground black pepper in a food processor or blender.

3 Serve swirled with a little yogurt, some toasted cumin seeds and a little torn mint.

PER SERVING 90 kcals, protein 6g, carbs 15g, fat 1g, sat fat none, fibre 4g, sugar 5g, salt 1.69g

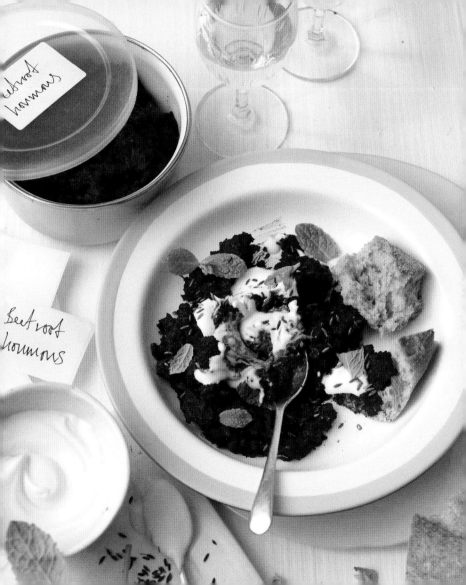

Beetroot
houmous

Spring greens with lemon dressing

As this dish cools and the veg soaks up the dressing, the greens will lose some of their vibrancy – but it will still taste good, so leftovers are worth saving for lunch.

53 KCALS

TAKES 15 MINUTES ● **SERVES 8**

250g/9oz broccoli,
thicker stalks halved
400g/14oz spring greens,
thick stalks removed
and shredded

FOR THE DRESSING
2 garlic cloves, crushed
zest and juice 1 lemon
2 tbsp olive oil

1 To make the dressing, mix the garlic, lemon juice and zest, olive oil and some seasoning together.
2 Bring a large pan of water to the boil, then add the broccoli and greens, and cook for about 5 minutes until tender.
3 Drain well, then toss through the dressing and serve.

PER SERVING 53 kcals, protein 3g, carbs 2g, fat 4g, sat fat 1g, fibre 3g, sugar 2g, salt none

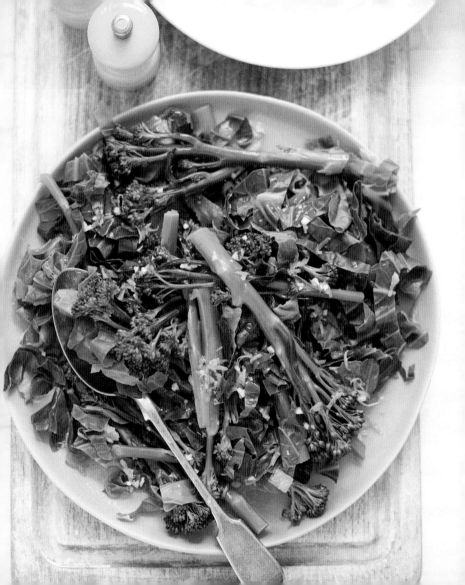

Smoked salmon & avocado sushi

Homemade sushi is much easier to make than you think, and the combination of protein and carbohydrates means just a couple of rolls will keep you full for a while.

49 KCALS

TAKES 30 MINUTES • MAKES 32

300g/10oz sushi rice

2 tbsp rice vinegar or white
  wine vinegar

1 tsp caster sugar

1 large avocado

juice ½ lemon

4 sheets nori seaweed

4 large slices smoked salmon

1 bunch chives

sweet soy sauce (kecap manis),
  for dipping

1 Put the rice in a small pan with 600ml/ 1 pint water. Bring to the boil and cook for 10 minutes until the water is absorbed and the rice is tender. Stir through the vinegar and sugar, then cover and cool.

2 Skin, stone and slice the avocado. Put in a bowl and squeeze over the lemon juice.

3 Divide the rice among the nori sheets and spread it out evenly, leaving a 1cm/ ½in border at the top and bottom. Lay the salmon over the rice, followed by lengths of chives, and finally position the avocado across the centre.

4 Fold the bottom edge of the seaweed over the filling, then roll it up firmly. Dampen the top border with a little water to help it seal the roll. Repeat to make four rolls. At this stage, the rolls can be wrapped individually in cling film and chilled until ready to serve.

5 Using a serrated knife, cut each roll into eight rounds. Serve with sweet soy sauce for dipping.

PER SUSHI 49 kcals, protein 2g, carbs 7g, fat 2g, sat fat none, fibre 1g, sugar none, salt 0.24g

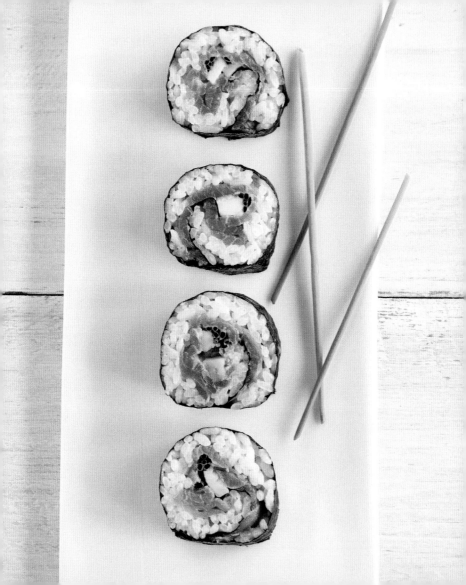

Honey-roasted swede with chilli

Swede can be roasted just like a potato, with the added advantage that it doesn't need boiling beforehand.

97 KCALS

TAKES 1 HOUR • SERVES 4

1 large swede, peeled and cut into
large chunks
2 tbsp olive oil
1 tbsp clear honey
1 tsp cumin seeds
1 large red chilli, deseeded
and chopped
small bunch coriander, chopped

1 Heat oven to 200°C/180°C fan/gas 6. Toss the swede in the olive oil in a shallow roasting tin, then season. Roast in the oven for 35–40 minutes, tossing occasionally, until the swede is golden and soft.

2 Stir in the honey and cumin seeds, and continue to roast for 10 minutes until just starting to catch. Remove and stir through the chilli and coriander to serve.

PER SERVING 97 kcals, protein 1g, carbs 10g, fat 6g, sat fat 1g, fibre 3g, sugar 10g, salt 0.1g

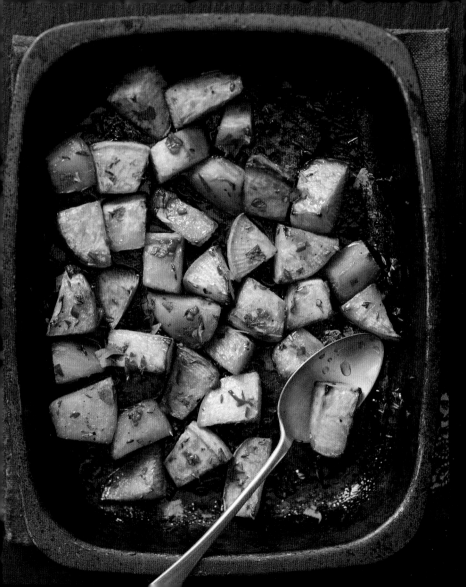

Ricotta & spring-onion dip

This dip takes only minutes to make and is great for a nibble before dinner or served at lunch with celery or cucumber sticks and some toasted wholemeal pitta or bread.

72 KCALS

TAKES 5 MINUTES
- **SERVES 6 AS A NIBBLE**

140g/5oz ricotta
3 spring onions, roughly chopped
juice and zest ½ lemon
50g/2oz soured cream, crème fraîche
  or natural yogurt

1 Whizz the ricotta with most of the chopped spring onions and the lemon juice and zest, soured cream, crème fraîche or natural yogurt and some seasoning.

2 Keep chilled until ready to eat, then scatter with the remaining sliced spring onions before serving.

PER SERVING 72 kcals, protein 3g, carbs 1g, fat 6g, sat fat 4g, fibre none, sugar 1g, salt 0.1g

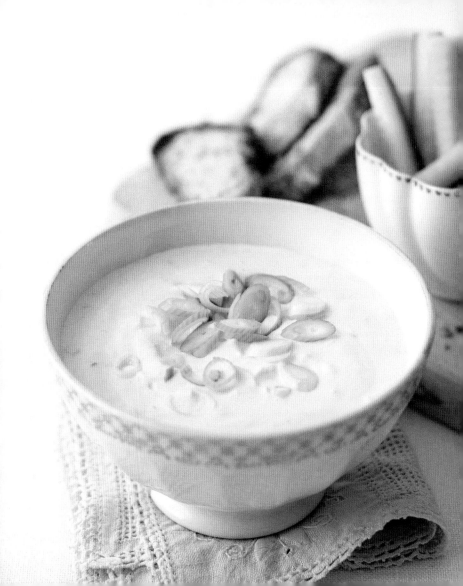

Warm chicken-liver salad

This really is a superfood salad – a good source of iron, folic acid and vitamin C that's also low in fat. Tuck in!

83 KCALS

TAKES 25 MINUTES • SERVES 4

140g/5oz fine green beans
200g/7oz chicken livers, trimmed
½ tbsp olive oil
½ tsp chopped fresh or dried
    rosemary leaves
1 whole chicory or Baby Gem lettuce,
    separated into leaves
100g/4oz watercress
3 tbsp balsamic vinegar

1 Cook the green beans in a pan of boiling water for 3 minutes, drain and keep warm. Meanwhile, toss together the chicken livers, olive oil and rosemary. Heat a large non-stick pan and cook the chicken livers over a high heat for 5–6 minutes until nicely browned and cooked through – they should still be a little pink in the centre.

2 Arrange the beans on serving plates with the chicory or lettuce leaves and watercress. Add the vinegar to the pan, cook for a couple of seconds then spoon over the salad. Serve with crusty bread, if you like.

PER SERVING 83 kcals, protein 10g, carbs 4g, fat 3g, sat fat 1g, fibre 1g, sugar 3g, salt 0.13g

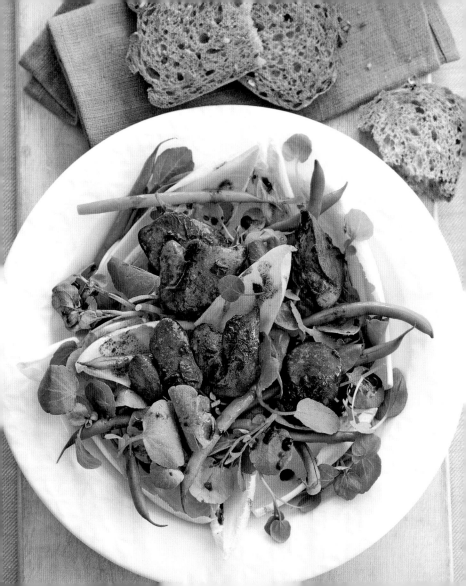

Hot & sour broth with prawns

This makes a lovely starter or lunch, and can be knocked up in 15 minutes. A handful of rice noodles will make it even more satisfying without adding too many calories.

93 KCALS

TAKES 15 MINUTES • SERVES 4

3 tbsp rice vinegar or white
   wine vinegar
500ml/18fl oz chicken stock
1 tbsp light soy sauce
1–2 tbsp golden caster sugar
thumb-sized piece of fresh ginger,
   peeled and thinly sliced
2 small hot red chillies, deseeded
   and thinly sliced
3 spring onions, thinly sliced
300g/10oz small raw peeled prawns

1 Put the vinegar, stock, soy sauce, sugar (start with 1 tablespoon and add the second at the end if you want the soup sweeter), ginger, chillies and spring onions in a pan and bring to a simmer.
2 Cook for 1 minute, then add the prawns to heat through. Serve in small bowls or cups.

PER SERVING 93 kcals, protein 17g, carbs 5g, fat 1g, sat fat none, fibre none, sugar 5g, salt 1.39g

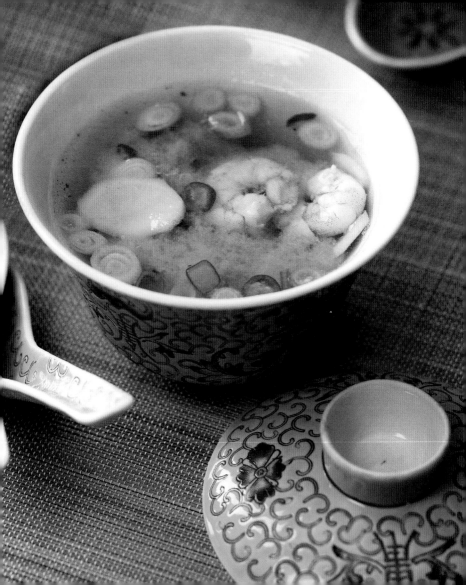

Tomato & onion salad

It's really worth waiting for summer to make this salad, because then the flavours of the tomatoes in the shops will be so much better.

53 KCALS

TAKES 15 MINUTES • SERVES 8

1kg/2lb 4oz mixed tomatoes,
    some large, some cherry
1 red onion, finely chopped

FOR THE DRESSING

2 tbsp wholegrain mustard
2 tbsp sherry vinegar
2 tbsp clear honey

1 Wash the tomatoes and cut each to roughly the same size – halve any cherry tomatoes and chunkily dice or wedge any big ones. Stir in the red onion.

2 Whisk together the mustard, sherry vinegar and honey for the dressing with some seasoning. Stir through the dressing up to 2 hours ahead of serving.

PER SERVING 53 kcals, protein 1g, carbs 9g, fat 1g, sat fat none, fibre 2g, sugar 9g, salt 0.2g

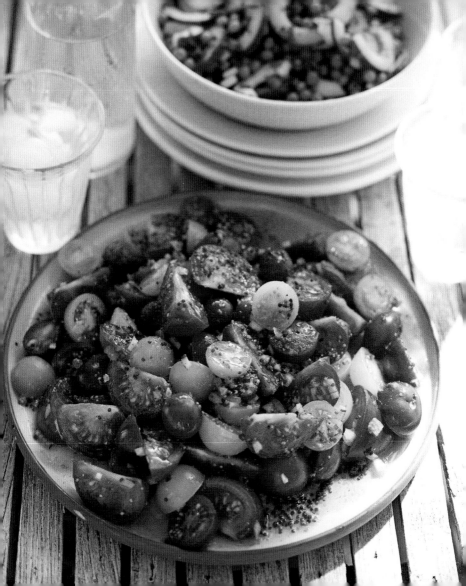

Healthier sausage rolls

You'll love these healthy versions of a party favourite – still melt-in-the-mouth but containing just half the fat of the classic recipe.

99 KCALS

TAKES 45 MINUTES, PLUS CHILLING

● **MAKES 16**

FOR THE FILLING

1 plump shallot, finely chopped

1 tsp rapeseed oil

100g/4oz green lentils, drained weight
    from a 400g can

300g/10oz lean pork mince (8% fat),
    preferably organic

50g/2oz fresh white breadcrumbs

2 tsp finely chopped tarragon leaves

good pinch dry mustard powder

good pinch grated nutmeg

FOR THE PASTRY

flour, for dusting

½ x 375g sheet ready-rolled
    puff pastry

2 tsp semi-skimmed milk,
    to seal and glaze

1 Heat oven to 220°C/200°C fan/gas 7 and line a baking sheet with baking parchment.

2 Fry the shallot in the oil until soft. Cool. Mash the lentils in a bowl, then stir in the rest of the filling ingredients, the shallot, a small pinch of salt and a good grinding of black pepper. Chill for 20 minutes.

3 Halve the filling. Lightly flour the work surface and roll each half, one at a time, into a 28cm/11¼in-long sausage shape.

4 Roll out the pastry on a clean, lightly floured work surface to a 28cm/11¼in square. Cut in half to give two rectangles. Lay one of the sausage shapes along a long edge of one pastry. Roll the pastry around it almost to enclose, then brush a little milk down the opposite long side. Roll the join underneath and seal. Slice into eight rolls. Put on the prepared baking sheet, with the joins underneath. Make three indents on top of each roll. Repeat with the remaining pastry and filling. Brush the tops with milk.

5 Bake for 18–20 minutes until golden. Cool on a wire rack. Serve warm or cold.

PER ROLL 99 kcals, protein 6g, carbs 7g, fat 6g, sat fat 2g, fibre 1g, sugar 0.3g, salt 0.27g

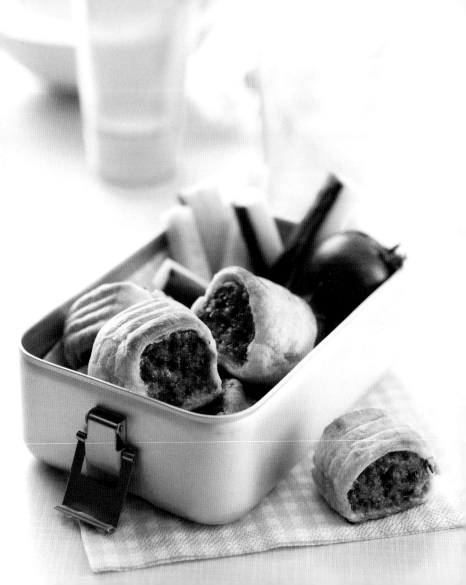

Festive red salad

This salad will keep for 3–4 days in the fridge, so it is really worth making a big batch and nibbling on it whenever you feel hungry.

93 KCALS

TAKES 20 MINUTES ● SERVES 15

1 red cabbage (about 650g/1lb 7oz)
2 small red onions, diced
2 red apples, cored and diced
250g pack cooked beetroot, diced
50g/2oz walnut pieces, roughly
    chopped
2 large oranges
5 tbsp red wine vinegar
3 tbsp redcurrant jelly
2 tbsp clear honey
2 tbsp olive oil

1 Quarter the cabbage, then cut out the white core at the bottom and discard. Finely shred the cabbage and tip into a large mixing bowl with the onions, apples, beetroot and walnuts. Finely grate over the zest from the oranges.
2 Cut a little from the top and bottom of each orange, so they sit flat on your work surface. Use a small serrated knife to cut away the peel and pith in strips down the orange. Holding each orange over a bowl, cut away the segments, letting them and any juice drop into the bowl. Squeeze any juice left in the membranes into the bowl too. Fish out the segments, roughly chop and add to the salad.
3 Whisk the red wine vinegar, redcurrant jelly, honey and oil into the orange juice with some seasoning, then stir into the salad.

PER SERVING 93 kcals, protein 2g, carbs 12g, fat 4g, sat fat 1g, fibre 3g, sugar 12g, salt 0.1g

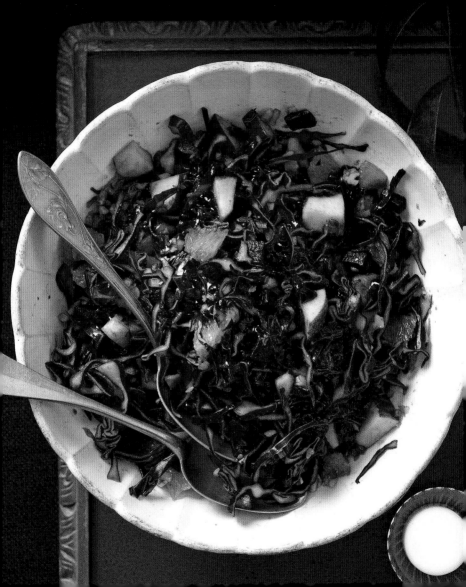

Thai-spiced turkey patties with noodle salad

Turkey is incredibly good for you, and its mild flavour means it can take a lot of spicing up. Make these low-fat patties for your family – the kids will love them too.

173 KCALS

TAKES 25 MINUTES ● **SERVES 4**

400g/14oz skinless turkey breast or
    fillet, roughly chopped
1 lemon grass stalk, finely chopped
2 garlic cloves, crushed
zest and juice 1 lime
3 tbsp low-sodium light soy sauce
small bunch coriander, chopped
1 red chilli, deseeded and chopped
2 nests medium wholewheat noodles
300g pack mixed pepper
    stir-fry vegetables

1 Heat the grill to medium-high. Put the turkey in a food processor and pulse until minced. Add the lemon grass, garlic and lime zest, and half the soy sauce, coriander and chilli, then pulse again until combined. Tip the mix into a bowl and add some black pepper. Shape into eight patties, then transfer to a non-stick baking sheet and grill for 3–4 minutes each side, until cooked through.

2 Meanwhile, soak the noodles according to the pack instructions, then drain and add the vegetables, the remaining soy sauce and the lime juice. Toss well, divide among plates and sprinkle with the remaining coriander and chilli. Serve with the turkey patties and some sweet chilli sauce for dipping, if you like.

PER SERVING 173 kcals, protein 27g, carbs 14g, fat 2g, sat fat none, fibre 2g, sugar 5g, salt 1.48g

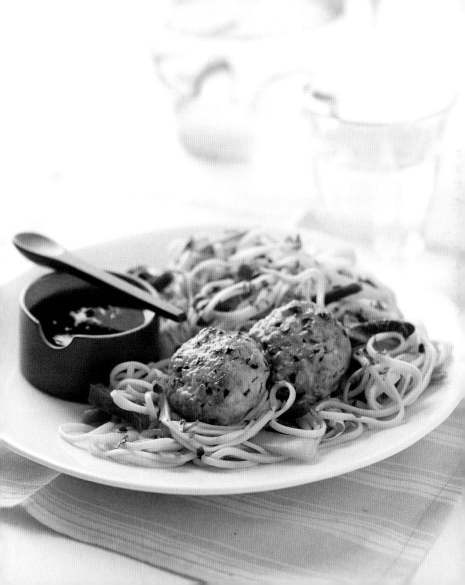

Crab & sweetcorn chowder

This quick soup is delicious all year round, but in summertime swap the frozen corn for fresh niblets, sliced straight off the cob.

191 KCALS

TAKES 35 MINUTES • SERVES 4

1 onion, finely chopped

1 leek, green and white parts
separated and sliced

2 carrots, chopped

850ml–1 litre/1½ pints–1¾ pints low-
sodium chicken or vegetable stock

1 large potato, peeled and diced

175g/6oz frozen sweetcorn

170g can white crabmeat, drained

4 tbsp light crème fraîche

1 tsp snipped chives

1 Put the onion, the white part of the leek and the carrots in a large pan, and pour on a few tablespoons of the stock. Cook over a medium heat for about 10 minutes, stirring regularly until soft. Add a splash more stock if the vegetables start to stick.
2 Add the potato, green leek parts and most of the stock, and simmer for 10–15 minutes, until the potato is tender.
3 Tip in the sweetcorn and crabmeat, then cook for a further 1–2 minutes. Remove from the heat and stir in the crème fraîche and some seasoning. Add the rest of the stock if the soup is too thick. Sprinkle with the chives and serve with brown bread, if you like.

PER SERVING 191 kcals, protein 13g, carbs 25g, fat 5g, sat fat 2g, fibre 3g, sugar 7g, salt 0.68g

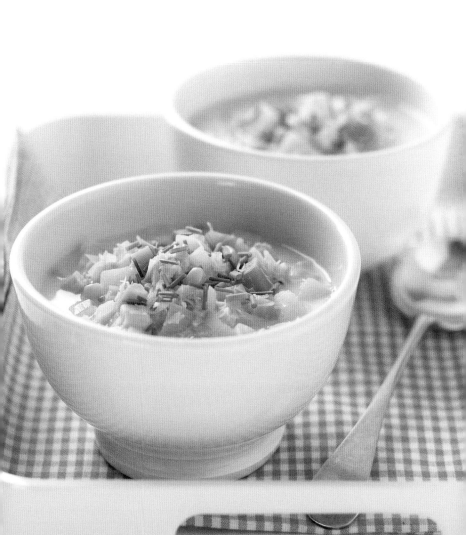

Chicken with harissa & tomatoes

This simple tray bake is packed with flavour. Serve with a crunchy green salad, boiled new potatoes and a spoonful of low-fat tzatziki.

184 KCALS

TAKES 17 MINUTES ● **SERVES 4**

4 boneless skinless chicken breasts

2 tsp harissa paste

1 tsp olive oil

1 tsp dried oregano

250g pack cherry tomatoes

handful olives (we used Kalamata)

1 Heat oven to 200°C/180°C fan/gas 6. Put the chicken into a medium roasting tin, then rub with the harissa, oil and oregano. Cover with foil and roast for 5 minutes, then remove the foil and add the cherry tomatoes and olives to the tin.

2 Roast for 10 minutes more until the tomato skins start to split and the chicken is cooked through, then serve.

PER SERVING 184 kcals, protein 34g, carbs 2g, fat 4g, sat fat 1g, fibre 1g, sugar 2g, salt 0.41g

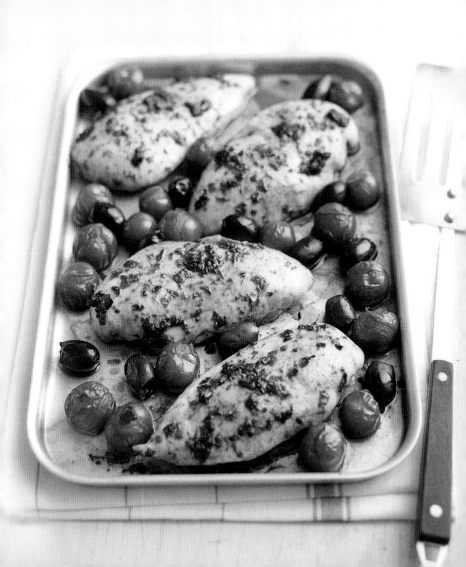

Green cucumber & mint gazpacho

This superhealthy chilled soup is packed with vegetables and full of flavour – perfect for a girls lunch in the garden.

186 KCALS

TAKES 20 MINUTES, PLUS CHILLING
- **SERVES 2**

1 cucumber, halved lengthways, deseeded and roughly chopped

1 yellow pepper, deseeded and roughly chopped

2 garlic cloves, crushed

1 small avocado, chopped

bunch spring onions, chopped

small bunch mint, chopped, plus extra to garnish (optional)

150g pot fat-free natural yogurt, plus extra to garnish (optional)

2 tbsp white wine vinegar, plus extra to taste

few shakes green Tabasco sauce, plus extra to taste

snipped chives and ice cubes, to garnish and serve (optional)

1 In a food processor or blender, blitz all the ingredients, reserving half the mint and yogurt, until smooth. Add a little extra vinegar, Tabasco and seasoning to taste, then add a splash of water if you like it thinner.

2 Chill until very cold, then serve with a dollop more yogurt, mint, chives and a few ice cubes, if you like. The soup will keep in the fridge for 2 days – just give it a good stir before serving.

PER SERVING 186 kcals, protein 8g, carbs 15g, fat 11g, sat fat 2g, fibre 5g, sugar 14g, salt 0.28g

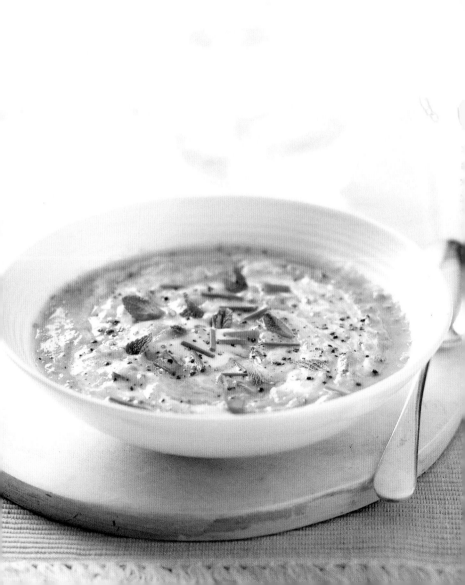

Caesar turkey burgers

Look for turkey-breast mince rather than thigh mince, as it's even lower in fat and calories.

199 KCALS

TAKES 35 MINUTES ● **SERVES 4**

1 garlic clove, crushed
1 anchovy fillet in olive oil, drained
    and diced (optional)
juice of 1 lemon
small bunch parsley, finely chopped
3 tbsp grated Parmesan
3 tbsp low-fat Greek yogurt
500g pack lean turkey mince
1 onion, finely chopped
1 romaine lettuce, shredded
4 small wholemeal buns
2 tomatoes, sliced

1 Heat oven to 200°C/180°C fan/gas 6. Mix together the garlic, anchovy, lemon juice, two-thirds of the Parmesan and the parsley. Put half in a small bowl, mix with the yogurt and set aside. Mix the other half in a large bowl with the mince and onion, then season. Shape into four burgers and put in a roasting tin, then cook for 15–20 minutes, until cooked through.
2 Meanwhile, toss the lettuce with the yogurt dressing and slice the buns.
3 To assemble, put the burgers in the buns with some salad and a few tomato slices. Serve the burgers with any leftover salad sprinkled with the reserved Parmesan.

PER SERVING 199 kcals, protein 12g, carbs 28g, fat 5g, sat fat 2g, fibre 4g, sugar 6g, salt 0.81g

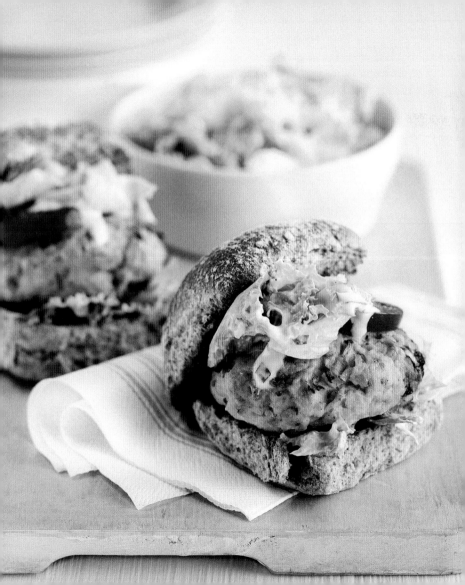

Saucy prawns

Just as tasty as a Chinese takeaway, but with only a percentage of the fat – so you can enjoy this every Friday guilt-free!

127 KCALS

TAKES 20 MINUTES ● **SERVES 1**

1 garlic clove, crushed
juice of ½ lemon, plus wedges
    to garnish
1 tbsp low-sugar and -salt
    tomato ketchup
100ml/3½fl oz chicken stock (from a
    cube is fine)
100g/4oz large cooked, peeled prawns
steamed broccoli and rice, to serve

1 Heat the garlic, lemon juice, ketchup and stock together in a frying pan. Simmer until syrupy and thickened.
2 Add the prawns and some seasoning, then heat through. Serve with some steamed broccoli, rice and the lemon wedges, if you like.

PER SERVING 127 kcals, protein 26g, carbs 4g, fat 1g, sat fat none, fibre 1g, sugar 3g, salt 2.30g

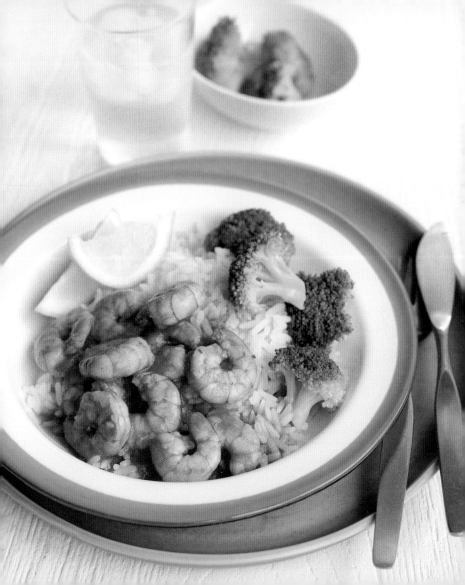

Thai squash soup

This gorgeous soup is really low in fat, but if you can find light coconut milk you'll make it even healthier!

161 KCALS

TAKES 35 MINUTES • SERVES 4

1 onion, chopped

1 lemon grass stalk, bashed
  and shredded

1–2 red chillies, deseeded and
  roughly chopped

1kg/2.2lb butternut squash, peeled
  and diced

juice of 1 lime

125ml/4fl oz coconut milk

small bunch coriander, leaves picked,
  to garnish

1 Fry the onion, lemon grass and most of the chilli in a large pan with a splash of water for 2–3 minutes until softened – add more water if it starts to catch. Tip in the squash and stir. Cover with 1 litre/1¾ pints water, bring to the boil and simmer for 15 minutes until the squash is tender. Add the lime juice then remove from the heat and blitz with a hand blender until smooth.

2 Pour in the coconut milk, season, then return to the heat gently to warm through. Ladle into bowls and serve sprinkled with coriander and the remaining chilli.

PER SERVING 161 kcals, protein 4g, carbs 23g, fat 6g, sat fat 5g, fibre 5g, sugar 13g, salt none

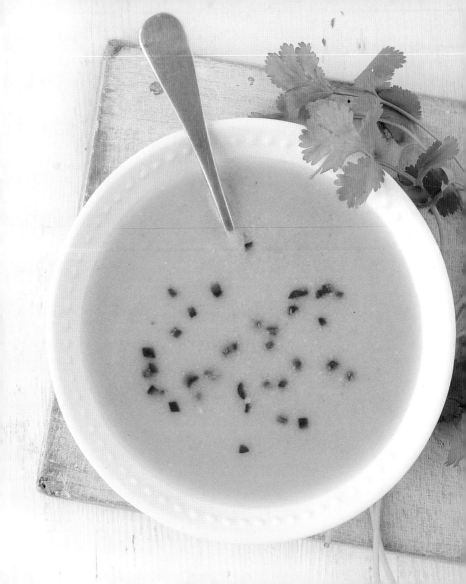

Stuffed marrow bake

Kids will love this tasty bake. Why not serve it with some light mashed potatoes – simply mash them with some milk instead of butter or cream.

198 KCALS

TAKES 1 HOUR ● SERVES 6

1 tbsp olive oil
1 onion, chopped
1 garlic clove, crushed
1 tbsp dried mixed herbs
500g pack turkey mince
2 x 400g cans chopped tomatoes
1 marrow
4 tbsp breadcrumbs
3 tbsp grated Parmesan

1 Heat oven to 200°C/180°C fan/gas 6. Heat the oil in a large frying pan and cook the onion, garlic and 2 teaspoons of the herbs for 3 minutes until starting to soften. Add the turkey and brown all over, then tip in the tomatoes and cook for 5 minutes more.

2 Cut the marrow in half, scoop out the middle of the marrow then discard (or fry, then freeze for another time – try it mashed with potato) and cut into 4cm/1½in-thick slices. Arrange the slices in a baking dish. Spoon the mince into the middle of each marrow slice, then spoon the rest over the top. Cover with foil and bake for 30 minutes.

3 Meanwhile, mix the remaining herbs with the breadcrumbs and Parmesan. Remove the marrow from the oven, uncover and sprinkle over the crumbs. Return to the oven for 10 minutes more, uncovered, until the crumbs are golden and crisp and the marrow is tender.

PER SERVING 198 kcals, protein 24g, carbs 15g, fat 5g, sat fat 2g, fibre 3g, sugar 8g, salt 0.55g

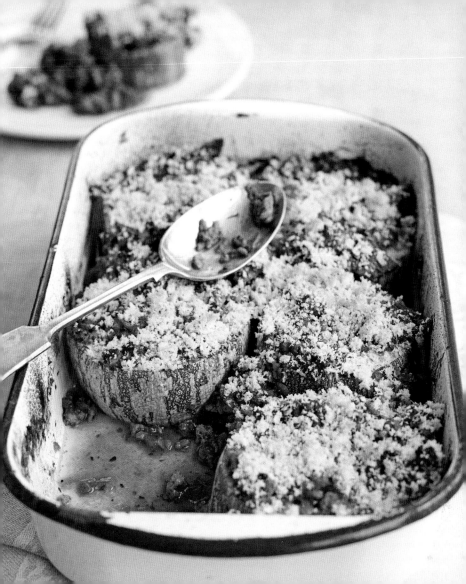

Charred aubergine, pepper & bulgar salad

A great summer lunch, or serve this as an accompaniment to a grilled chicken breast, small salmon fillet or lean fillet steak for dinner.

198 KCALS

TAKES 20 MINUTES • SERVES 4

175g/6oz bulgar wheat
2 tbsp sundried tomato paste
4 baby aubergines, each sliced
    lengthways into 3
1 red pepper, sliced into
    1cm-/½in-thick slices
2 tsp olive oil
handful basil leaves

1 Prepare the bulgar according to the pack instructions. Tip into a large bowl and stir through the tomato paste. Season well.
2 Heat a barbecue or griddle pan. Drizzle the aubergines and red pepper with the oil and cook for 5 minutes on each side until lightly charred.
3 Stir the aubergines and red pepper into the bulgar mixture, then season and stir through the basil and serve.

PER SERVING 198 kcals, protein 6g, carbs 38g, fat 3g, sat fat none, fibre 6g, sugar 6g, salt 0.2g

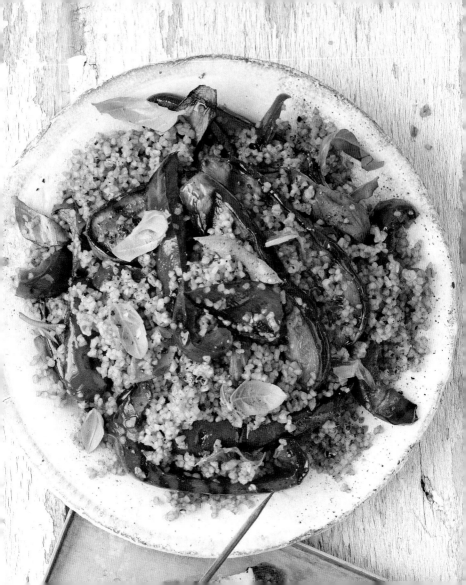

Spicy harissa, aubergine & chickpea soup

Harissa is a fragrant, spiced paste – if you don't like your food so spicy, add a spoon of fat-free Greek yogurt to the soup bowls as you serve.

157 KCALS

TAKES 50 MINUTES ● SERVES 4

1 onion, chopped
1 tbsp olive oil
2 tbsp harissa paste
2 aubergines, diced
400g can chopped tomatoes
400g can chickpeas, drained
   and rinsed
2 tbsp chopped coriander leaves

1 Soften the onion in the oil in a large pan. Add the harissa and cook for 2 minutes, stirring. Add the aubergine and coat in the harissa.

2 Add the chopped tomatoes, chickpeas and 500ml/18fl oz water. Bring to the boil and simmer for 30 minutes.

3 Stir through the chopped coriander, season and serve.

PER SERVING 157 kcals, protein 6g, carbs 20g, fat 5g, sat fat 1g, fibre 9g, sugar 8g, salt 0.7g

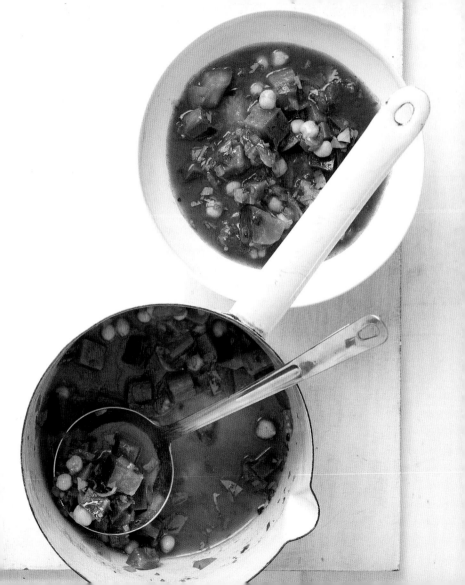

Veggie breakfast bakes

Who says being on a diet means you have to give up your cooked breakfast? Add a
low-fat sausage or some rashers of turkey bacon to make this meaty, but still healthy.

127 KCALS

TAKES 45 MINUTES ● SERVES 4

4 large field mushrooms
8 tomatoes, halved
1 garlic clove, thinly sliced
2 tsp olive oil
200g bag spinach leaves
4 eggs

1 Heat oven to 200°C/180°C fan/gas 6. Put the mushrooms and tomatoes into four ovenproof dishes. Divide the garlic among the dishes, drizzle over the oil and some seasoning, then bake for 10 minutes.

2 Meanwhile, put the spinach into a large colander, then pour over a kettle of boiling water to wilt it. Squeeze out any excess water, then add the spinach to the dishes.

3 Make a little gap between the vegetables and crack an egg into each dish. Return to the oven and cook for a further 8–10 minutes or until the egg is cooked to your liking.

PER SERVING 127 kcals, protein 9g, carbs 5g, fat 8g, sat fat 2g, fibre 3g, sugar 5g, salt 0.4g

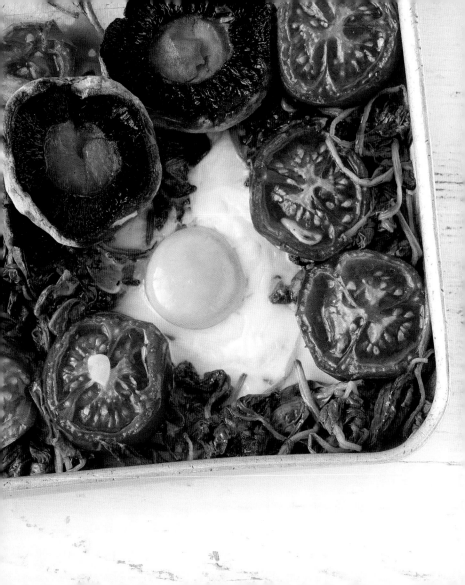

Pork & bulgar-stuffed peppers

Peppers are often much better value if you buy them in multi-packs of varying colours.

185 KCALS

TAKES 40 MINUTES • **SERVES 4**

4 peppers, halved and cores removed
200g/7oz pork mince
1 garlic clove, crushed
2 tsp ground cumin
1 tsp paprika
50g/2oz bulgar wheat
250ml/9fl oz vegetable stock
½ small bunch parsley, chopped
4 tbsp fat-free Greek yogurt, to serve

1 Put the peppers, cut-side down, on a plate and microwave on High for 4 minutes until cooked through (but not so soft they collapse). If they need longer, microwave for 1 minute more and repeat until done.

2 Put the pork in a cold frying pan and turn on the heat. Fry, breaking up any lumps, until it starts to brown. Stir in the garlic and spices for 1 minute, then add the bulgar and stock. Cover and simmer for 10 minutes until the bulgar is soft.

3 Heat the grill to medium-high. Stir half the parsley into the bulgar, then stuff into the peppers and set on a baking sheet. Grill to crisp, sprinkle over most of the remaining parsley, then serve with the yogurt mixed with the rest of the parsley.

PER SERVING 185 kcals, protein 13g, carbs 20g, fat 6g, sat fat 2g, fibre 3g, sugar 9g, salt 0.26g

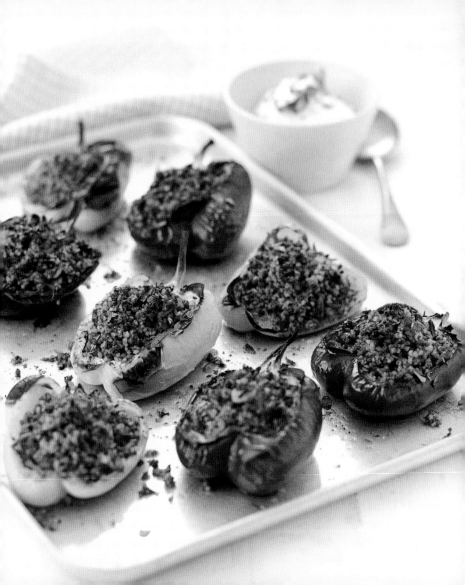

Mediterranean vegetables with lamb

This is a great summer stew; serve it with couscous, rice or even jacket potatoes.

192 KCALS

TAKES 45 MINUTES • SERVES 4

1 tbsp olive oil

250g/9oz lean lamb fillet, trimmed of
any fat and thinly sliced

140g/5oz shallots, halved

2 large courgettes, cut into chunks

½ tsp each ground cumin, paprika
and ground coriander

1 red, 1 orange and 1 green pepper,
deseeded and cut into chunks

1 garlic clove, sliced

150ml/¼ pint vegetable stock

250g/9oz cherry tomatoes

handful coriander leaves,
roughly chopped, to serve

1 Heat the oil in a large heavy-based frying pan. Cook the lamb and shallots over a high heat for 2–3 minutes until golden. Add the courgettes and stir-fry for 3–4 minutes until beginning to soften.

2 Add the spices and toss well, then add the peppers and garlic. Reduce the heat and cook over a moderate heat for 4–5 minutes until the peppers start to soften.

3 Pour in the stock and stir everything to coat. Add the tomatoes, season, then cover with a lid and simmer for 15 minutes, stirring occasionally, until the veg are tender. Stir through the coriander to serve.

PER SERVING 192 kcals, protein 17g, carbs 11g, fat 9g, sat fat 3g, fibre 4g, sugar 10g, salt 0.25g

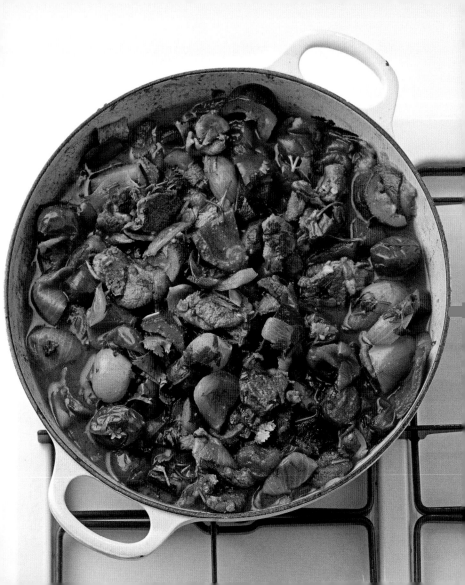

Teriyaki steak with fennel slaw

If there's only two of you, halve the number of steaks and marinade, but make the full quantity of slaw and keep it for lunch the following day.

188 KCALS

TAKES 20 MINUTES, PLUS
MARINATING • SERVES 4

2 tbsp reduced-salt dark soy sauce
1 tbsp red wine vinegar
1 tsp clear honey
4 sirloin or rump steaks, trimmed of all
   visible fat, each about 125g/4½oz

FOR THE FENNEL SLAW

1 large carrot, coarsely grated
1 fennel bulb, halved and thinly sliced
1 red onion, halved and thinly sliced
handful coriander leaves
juice 1 lime

1 Mix the soy, vinegar and honey in a dish, then add the steaks and leave to marinate for 10–15 minutes.

2 Toss together the carrot, fennel, onion and coriander for the slaw, then chill until ready to serve.

3 Remove the steaks from the marinade, reserving the marinade. Transfer the steaks to a hot griddle pan and cook for a few minutes on each side, depending on the thickness and how well done you like them. Set the meat aside to rest on a plate, then add the reserved marinade to the pan. Bubble the marinade until it reduces a little to make a sticky sauce.

4 Dress the salad with the lime juice, then pile on to plates and serve with the steaks. Spoon the sauce over the meat.

PER SERVING 188 kcals, protein 29g, carbs 7g, fat 5g, sat fat 2g, fibre 2g, sugar 6g, salt 1.05g

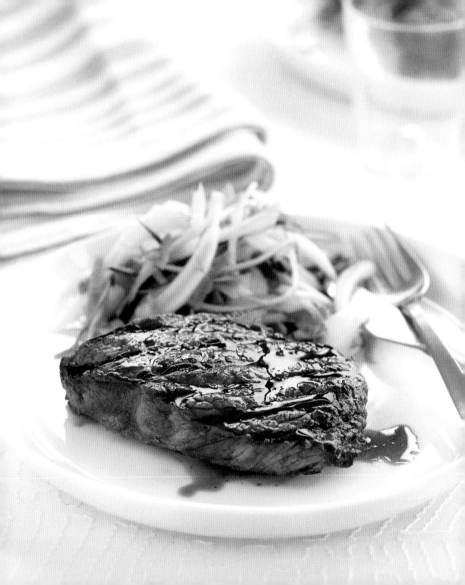

Prawn & mushroom five-spice stir-fry

No fancy ingredients here. this tasty stir-fry is full of simple things you'll find in any supermarket.

174 KCALS

TAKES 30 MINUTES • SERVES 4

2 tbsp sunflower oil

bunch spring onions, finely sliced

2 celery sticks, cut into matchsticks

1 garlic clove, crushed

½ tsp Chinese five-spice powder

2cm/1in piece ginger, grated

175g/6oz chestnut
   mushrooms, sliced

250g/9oz Savoy cabbage,
   finely shredded

450g/1lb raw peeled king prawns

4 tbsp low-salt light soy sauce

cooked wholewheat noodles, to serve

1 Heat the oil in a large frying pan or wok. Add the spring onions and celery and cook for a few minutes. Add the garlic, five-spice and ginger, and cook for 1 minute more. Add the mushrooms and cabbage and stir-fry for 5 minutes, until the cabbage has wilted.

2 Add the prawns and soy sauce, and cook for a further 5 minutes until the prawns are pink. Serve with wholewheat noodles, if you like.

PER SERVING 174 kcals, protein 23g, carbs 5g, fat 7g, sat fat 1g, fibre 4g, sugar 5g, salt 2.3g

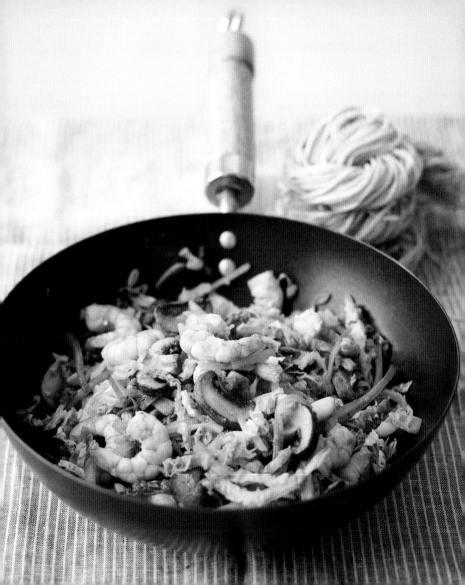

Spiced parsnip & cauliflower soup

This soup freezes beautifully, so make a double batch if your pans are big enough!

133 KCALS

TAKES 1 HOUR 5 MINUTES

● SERVES 6

1 tbsp olive oil

1 medium cauliflower, cut into florets

3 parsnips, peeled and chopped

2 onions, peeled and chopped

1 tbsp fennel seeds

1 tsp coriander seeds

½ tsp turmeric powder

3 garlic cloves, sliced

1–2 green chillies, deseeded
    and chopped

5cm/2in piece of fresh ginger, sliced

zest and juice 1 lemon, plus more
    juice to taste

1 litre/1¾ pints vegetable stock

handful coriander leaves, chopped

1 Heat the oil in a large pan and add the vegetables. Partially cover the pan and sweat the veg for 10–15 minutes until soft but not brown.

2 In a separate pan, dry-roast the spices with a pinch of salt for a few minutes until fragrant. Grind with a pestle and mortar to a fine powder.

3 Add the garlic, chilli, ginger and ground spices to the vegetables, and cook for about 5 minutes, stirring regularly. Add the lemon zest and juice. Pour in the stock, topping up if necessary just to cover the veg. Simmer for 25–30 minutes until all the vegetables are tender.

4 Purée with a blender until smooth. Dilute the consistency with more water if needed, until you get a thick but easily pourable soup. Season generously, stir in the coriander and add more lemon juice to balance the taste. Eat straight away or chill in the fridge to reheat. Finish with an extra grind of black pepper, to serve, if you like.

PER SERVING 133 kcals, protein 7g, carbs 18g, fat 4g, sat fat 1g, fibre 9g, sugar 11g, salt 0.6g

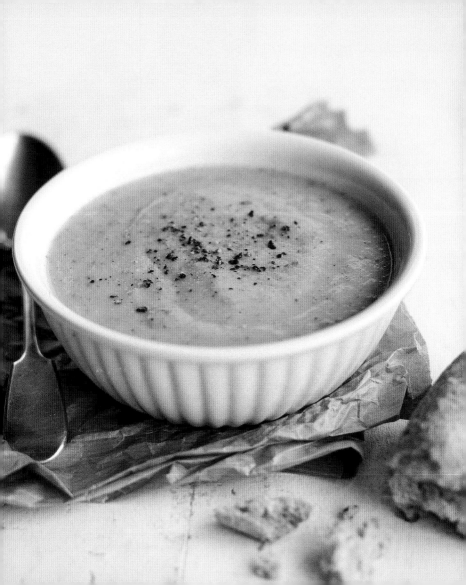

Creamy aubergine curry

Aubergines are filling and very low in calories, but they can be bland. Adding them to a curry is the perfect way to pep them up.

`190 KCALS`

TAKES 30 MINUTES ● **SERVES 4**

2 onions, roughly chopped
4cm/1½in piece ginger, chopped
4 tbsp toasted flaked almonds,
 plus 1 tbsp
1 tbsp curry powder
small bunch coriander, stalks and
 leaves separated
2 tsp olive oil
2 aubergines, chopped into
 large wedges
200g pot Greek yogurt

1 Whizz the onions, ginger, almonds, curry powder and coriander stalks until pulpy (add a splash of water if needed). Boil the kettle.

2 Heat the oil in a pan, then fry the aubergine for 5 minutes until browned. Scoop out and set aside. Add the onion paste to the pan, then cook for a few minutes, stirring, until softened. Return the aubergine to the pan with the yogurt and 400ml/15fl oz hot water. Stir, then simmer for 10–15 minutes until the aubergine is tender.

3 Season, then serve over basmati rice, scattered with the coriander leaves and extra almonds, if you like.

PER SERVING 190 kcals, protein 8g, carbs 11g, fat 13g, sat fat 4g, fibre 6g, sugar 8g, salt 0.15g

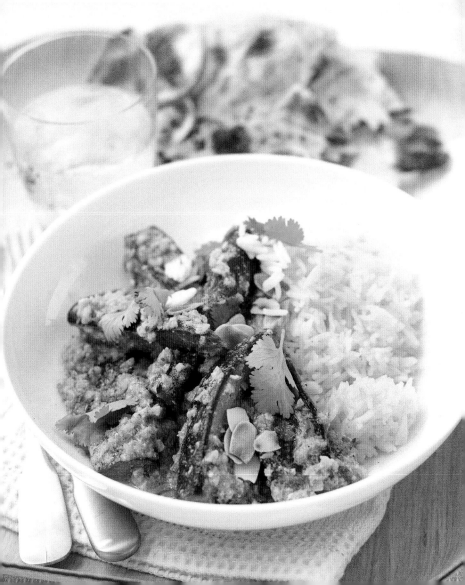

Summer eggs

Brunch, lunch or dinner – take your pick with this easy, flexible one-pan meal, and mop it up with warm crusty bread.

196 KCALS

TAKES 18 MINUTES • SERVES 2

1 tbsp olive oil

400g/14oz courgettes (about 2 large), chopped into small chunks

200g pack cherry tomatoes, halved

1 garlic clove, crushed

2 eggs

few basil leaves, to garnish

1 Heat the oil in a non-stick frying pan, then add the courgettes. Fry for 5 minutes, stirring every so often until they start to soften.

2 Add the tomatoes and garlic, then cook for a few minutes more. Stir in a little seasoning, then make two gaps in the mix and crack in the eggs.

3 Cover the pan with a lid or a sheet of foil, then cook for 2–3 minutes until the eggs are done to your liking. Scatter over a few basil leaves and serve with crusty bread, if you like.

PER SERVING 196 kcals, protein 12g, carbs 7g, fat 13g, sat fat 3g, fibre 3g, sugar 6g, salt 0.25g

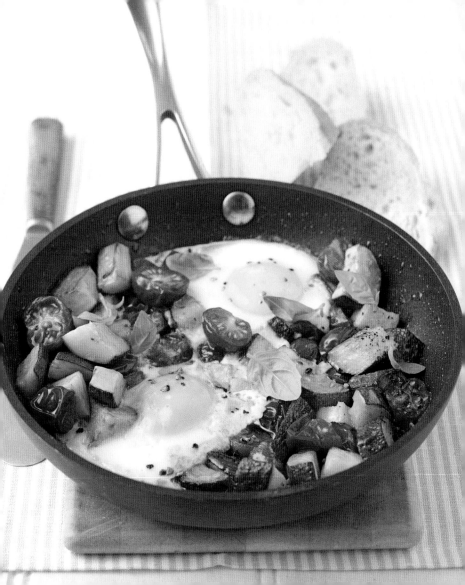

Asian chicken salad

Spicing up a low-calorie meal with some fresh hot chilli is a great way to make it feel more satisfying.

109 KCALS

TAKES 20 MINUTES ● **SERVES 2**

1 boneless, skinless chicken breast
1 tbsp Thai fish sauce
zest and juice ½ lime (about 1 tbsp)
1 tsp caster sugar
100g bag mixed leaves
large handful coriander leaves,
    roughly chopped
¼ red onion, thinly sliced
½ red chilli, deseeded and thinly sliced
¼ cucumber, sliced

1 Put the chicken in a pan and cover with cold water, bring to the boil, then cook for 10 minutes. Remove from the pan and tear into shreds.
2 To make the dressing, stir together the fish sauce, lime zest, juice and sugar in a small bowl until the sugar dissolves.
3 Put the leaves and coriander in a salad bowl, then top with the chicken, onion, chilli and cucumber. Pour the dressing over the salad and toss through when ready to eat.

PER SERVING 109 kcals, protein 19g, carbs 6g, fat 1g, sat fat none, fibre 1g, sugar 5g, salt 1.6g

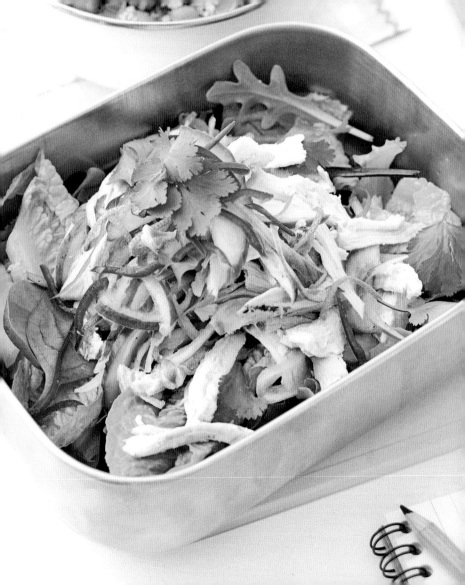

Open prawn-cocktail sandwich

Open sandwiches are a great option if you're trying to be healthy, as you can pile on the fillings so it feels really substantial.

173 KCALS

TAKES 15 MINUTES ● **SERVES 2**

2 tbsp extra-light mayonnaise
1 tbsp reduced-sugar tomato ketchup
2 tbsp chopped dill leaves
1 lemon, cut into 8 wedges
100g pack cooked and peeled
  North Atlantic prawns
½ cucumber, deseeded and diced
2 handfuls cherry tomatoes, halved
20g bag rocket leaves
2 thin slices wholemeal bread

1 Make the dressing in a medium bowl by mixing together the mayonnaise, ketchup, half the dill, the juice from 4 of the lemon wedges and some seasoning. Toss in the prawns, cucumber and tomatoes.
2 Arrange the bread on two plates, top each with rocket and pile on the prawn filling. Scatter with the remaining dill and serve with the remaining lemon wedges, for squeezing over.

PER SERVING 173 kcals, protein 17g, carbs 22g, fat 3g, sat fat none, fibre 3g, sugar 7g, salt 1.6g

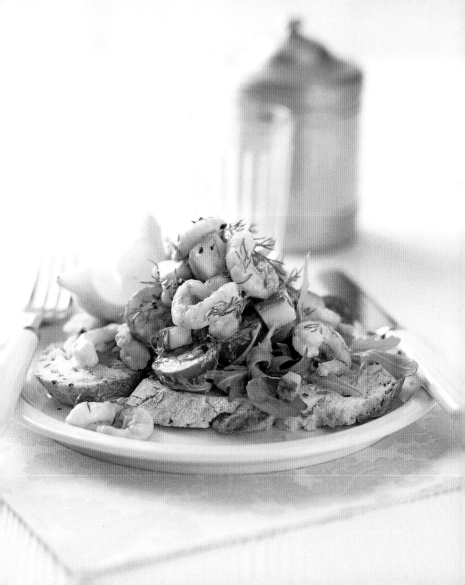

Steamed fish with ginger & spring onion

Serve these gorgeous fragrant parcels with brown basmati rice, rice noodles or mashed sweet potato.

145 KCALS

TAKES 30 MINUTES ● SERVES 4

100g/4oz pak choi
4 x 150g fillets firm white fish
5cm/2in piece ginger, finely shredded
2 garlic cloves, finely sliced
2 tbsp low-salt light soy sauce
1 tsp mirin or sweet rice wine
1 bunch spring onions, finely shredded
handful coriander leaves, chopped
1 lime, cut into wedges, to garnish

1 Heat oven to 200°C/180°C fan/gas 6. Cut a large rectangle of foil, big enough to make a large envelope. Put the pak choi on the foil, followed by the fish, then the ginger and garlic. Pour over the soy sauce and rice wine, then season.

2 Fold over the foil and seal the three edges, then put on a baking sheet. Cook for 20 minutes, open the parcel and scatter over the spring onions and coriander. Serve with lime wedges to squeeze over.

PER SERVING 145 kcals, protein 29g, carbs 4g, fat 1g, sat fat none, fibre 1g, sugar 3g, salt 1.1g

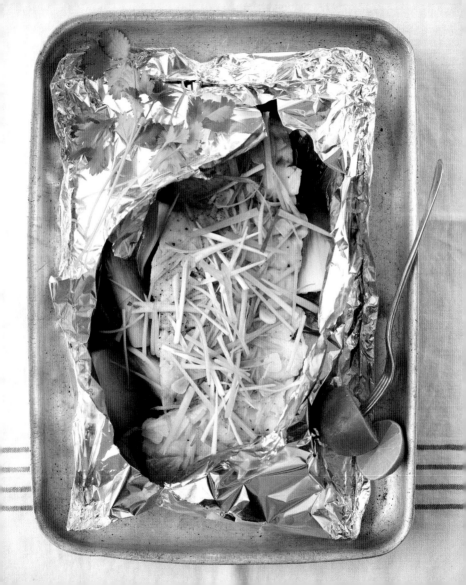

Ham & beetroot salad bowl

Make different versions of this salad by replacing the ham with any of the following: flaked smoked mackerel, peeled prawns or a little crumbled goat's cheese.

166 KCALS

TAKES 15 MINUTES ● **SERVES 2**

100g/4oz frozen peas
175g/6oz cooked beetroot
2 spring onions, thinly sliced
2 tbsp Greek yogurt
2 tsp horseradish sauce
½ iceberg lettuce, shredded
100g/4oz wafer-thin sliced ham, torn
    into strips

1 Pour boiling water over the peas and leave for 2 minutes, then drain well. Chop the beetroot into cubes.
2 Tip the peas, beetroot and spring onions into a bowl and mix well. In a small bowl, mix the yogurt and horseradish, then add about 1 tablespoon boiling water to make a pouring sauce.
3 Pile the lettuce into bowls, then spoon over the beetroot mix. Thinly drizzle the dressing over the salad and top with the ham.

PER SERVING 166 kcals, protein 16g, carbs 17g, fat 4g, sat fat 2g, fibre 5g, sugar 13g, salt 1.92g

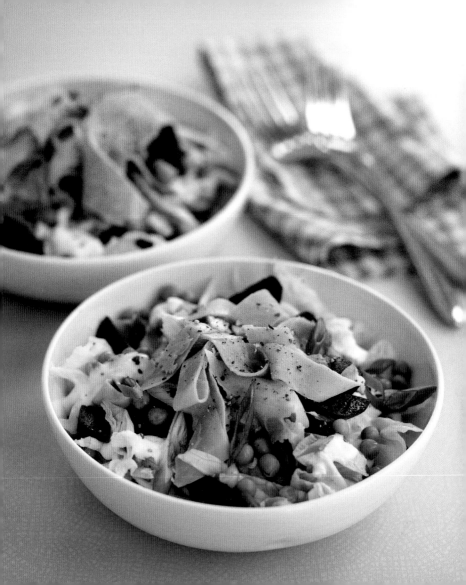

Pineapple, beef & ginger stir-fry

This unusual stir-fry is absolutely packed with flavour – buy small tubs of fresh, ready-prepared pineapple if you don't fancy dealing with a whole fruit.

267 KCALS

TAKES 25 MINUTES • SERVES 2

400g/14oz rump steak, thinly sliced

3 tbsp dark soy sauce

2 tbsp light soft brown sugar

1 tbsp chilli sauce

1 tbsp rice wine vinegar

2 tsp vegetable oil

thumb-sized piece of fresh ginger,
    cut into fine matchsticks

4 spring onions, cut into
    3cm/1¼in lengths

200g/7oz pineapple, cut into chunks

handful coriander leaves, to garnish

1 Mix the steak, soy sauce, sugar, chilli sauce and vinegar together, and set aside for 10 minutes.

2 Heat a wok with 1 teaspoon of the oil. Lift the steak from the marinade, reserving the marinade, and sear the steak, in batches, then remove. Add a bit more oil and fry the ginger until golden.

3 Add the spring onions and pineapple, and return the steak to the pan. Stir to heat through for 1 minute, then add the reserved marinade. Keep stirring until the marinade becomes thick and everything is hot. Serve sprinkled with coriander, and with rice and greens, if you like.

PER SERVING 267 kcals, protein 22g, carbs 18g, fat 12g, sat fat 5g, fibre 1g, sugar 18g, salt 2.4g

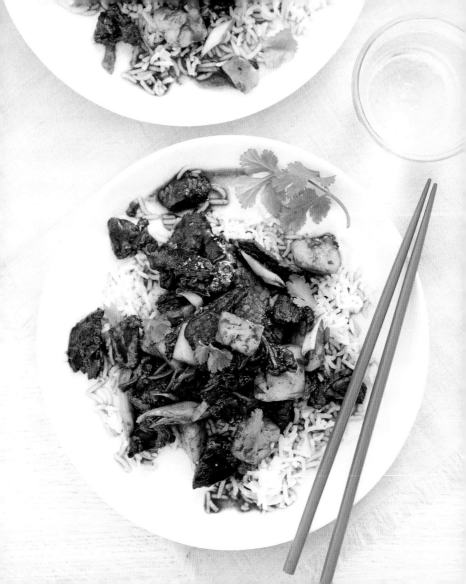

Low-fat chicken balti

You don't have to give up curries when you have this healthier recipe up your sleeve.

217 KCALS

TAKES 1 HOUR, PLUS MARINATING

● **SERVES 4**

450g/1lb boneless skinless chicken breasts, cut into bite-sized pieces

1 tbsp lime juice

1 tsp each paprika, cumin seeds, tumeric, ground cumin, ground coriander and garam masala

¼ tsp hot chilli powder

1½ tbsp sunflower or groundnut oil

1 cinnamon stick

3 cardamom pods, split

1 small–medium green chilli

1 onion, coarsely grated

2 garlic cloves, very finely chopped

2.5cm/1in piece ginger, grated

250ml/9fl oz organic passata

1 red pepper, deseeded and cut into small chunks

1 medium tomato, chopped

85g/3oz baby leaf spinach

handful coriander leaves, to garnish

1 Mix the chicken with the lime juice, paprika, chilli powder and a grinding of black pepper. Marinate for 15 minutes.

2 Heat 1 tablespoon of the oil in a large non-stick pan. Add the cinnamon stick, cardamom pods, whole chilli and cumin seeds and stir-fry briefly. Stir in the onion, garlic and ginger and fry until the onion starts to brown. Add the remaining oil and chicken and fry until it no longer looks raw. Stir in the turmeric, ground cumin, ground coriander and garam masala for 2 minutes.

3 Pour in the passata and 150ml/¼ pint water, then drop in the chunks of pepper. When starting to bubble, lower the heat and simmer for 15–20 minutes or until the chicken is tender.

4 Stir in the tomato, simmer for 3 minutes, then add the spinach and season. If you want to thin down the sauce, splash in a little more water. Scatter with fresh coriander and serve with chapatis or basmati rice, if you like.

PER SERVING 217 kcals, protein 30g, carbs 10g, fat 7g, sat fat 1g, fibre 3g, sugar 8g, salt 0.5g

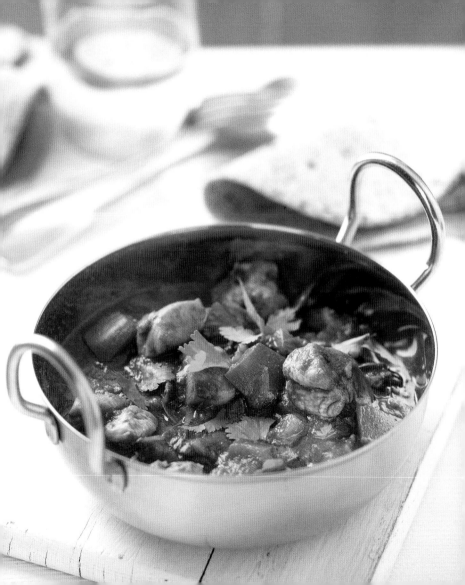

Cheesy bean & sweetcorn cakes with salsa

A vibrant Tex-Mex mix with a difference – it's good for you! Just make sure you use a strong Cheddar; that way a little adds a lot of flavour.

292 KCALS

TAKES 30 MINUTES • SERVES 4

400g can mixed beans in water,
   drained and rinsed
400g can chickpeas, drained and rinsed
50g/2oz mature Cheddar, grated
198g can sweetcorn, drained
   and rinsed
8 jalapeño slices from a jar,
   finely chopped
1 egg, beaten
small handful coriander
   leaves, chopped
2 tbsp vegetable oil
10 cherry tomatoes, quartered
½ red onion, sliced
juice ½ lime

1 Put the beans and chickpeas in the bowl of a food processor and blend until smooth. Tip into a bowl and add the cheese, sweetcorn, jalapeños, egg and half the coriander. Season, mix well to combine, then shape into eight patties.

2 Heat the oil in a large frying pan and cook the patties for 4 minutes on each side – you may have to do this in batches. Keep them warm in the oven as you go.

3 Mix the tomatoes, onion, remaining coriander and lime juice with a little salt to make a salsa. Serve the cakes with the salsa and some salad leaves, if you like.

PER SERVING 292 kcals, protein 17g, carbs 24g, fat 13g, sat fat 4g, fibre 12g, sugar 2g, salt 1.9g

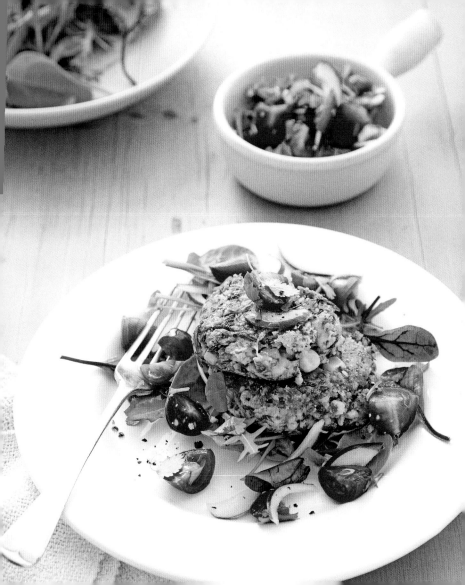

Beef & bacon meatloaf

With just five ingredients, this meatloaf makes a great budget supper for the family. You could even serve it for Sunday lunch!

240 KCAL

TAKES 50 MINUTES • **SERVES 6**

sunflower oil, for greasing
85g pack sage and onion stuffing mix
1 beef stock cube
8 rashers rindless smoked
   streaky bacon
500g pack beef mince (use one with
   less than 20% fat)

1 Heat oven to 180°C/160°C fan/gas 4 and oil the inside of a 900g/2lb loaf tin. Tip the stuffing mix into a bowl, crumble in the stock cube and pour over 300ml/½ pint boiling water. Give it a good stir, then set aside.

2 Stretch the bacon rashers a little by running the back of a spoon along their length, then use 6–7 to line the base and longest sides of the tin. Chop the rest.

3 Mix the chopped bacon and mince into the stuffing with some black pepper, then press into the bacon-lined tin and bake for 40 minutes until firm. Turn out and serve sliced.

PER SERVING 240 kcals, protein 23g, carbs 3g, fat 15g, sat fat 6g, fibre none, sugar none, salt 1.6g

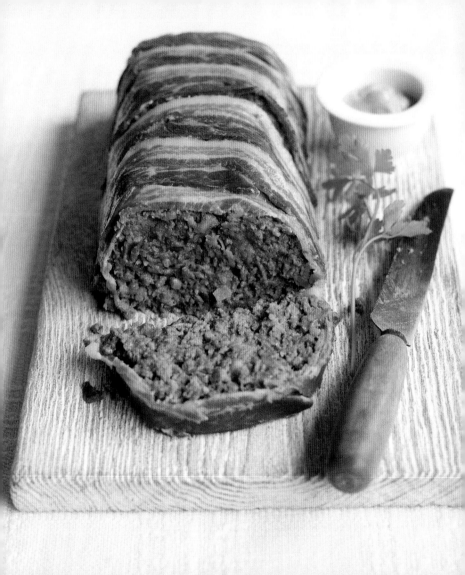

Thai fried rice with prawns & peas

All the satisfaction of a big bowl of pad Thai but with better-for-you brown rice and veg.

287 KCALS

TAKES 20 MINUTES • SERVES 4

2 tbsp vegetable oil

1 red onion, halved and sliced

2 garlic cloves, sliced

1 red chilli, deseeded and sliced

250g/9oz large raw peeled prawns

300g/10oz cooked brown rice (about
140g/5oz uncooked rice)

75g/2½oz frozen peas

1 tbsp each dark soy sauce and
Thai fish sauce

small bunch coriander, roughly
chopped, plus a few leaves
to garnish

4 eggs

1 Heat 1 tablespoon of the oil in a wok, add the onion, garlic and chilli and cook for 2–3 minutes until golden. Add the prawns and cook for 1 minute.

2 Tip in the rice and peas, and keep tossing until very hot. Add the soy and fish sauces, then stir through the chopped coriander. Keep warm while you fry the eggs.

3 Heat the remaining oil in a frying pan and fry the eggs with some seasoning. Divide the fried-rice mix among four bowls and top each with a fried egg. Serve scattered with coriander and some chilli sauce, if you like.

PER SERVING 287 kcals, protein 22g, carbs 21g, fat 12g, sat fat 3g, fibre 3g, sugar 3g, salt 1.9g

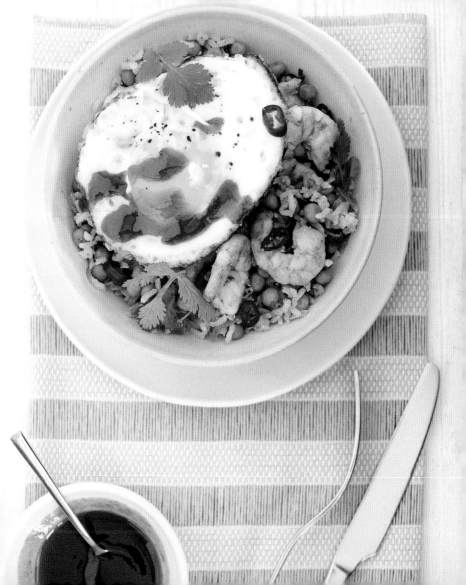

Courgette & quinoa-stuffed peppers

Use just five ingredients to create this healthy Mediterranean-style vegetarian supper for the family.

TAKES 30 MINUTES • SERVES 4

4 red peppers
1 tbsp olive oil, plus 1 tsp to fry
1 courgette, quartered lengthways and thinly sliced
2 x 250g packs ready-to-eat quinoa
85g/3oz feta, finely crumbled
handful parsley, roughly chopped

1 Heat oven to 200C/180C fan/gas 6. Cut each pepper in half through the stem and remove the seeds. Put the peppers, cut-side up, on a baking sheet, drizzle with the olive oil and season well. Roast for 15 minutes.

2 Meanwhile, heat the extra olive oil in a small frying pan, add the courgette and cook until soft. Remove from the heat, then stir through the quinoa, feta and parsley. Season with freshly ground black pepper.

3 Divide the quinoa mixture among the pepper halves, then return to the oven for 5 minutes to heat through.

PER SERVING 260 kcals, protein 11g, carbs 33g, fat 8g, sat fat 3g, fibre 11g, sugar 10g, salt 0.8g

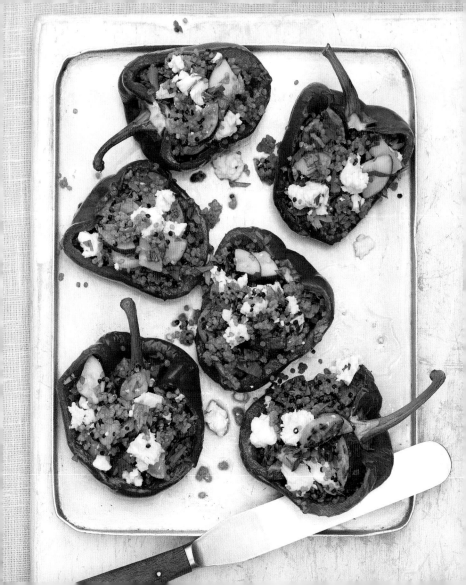

Curried carrot & butter bean soup

This low-fat but creamy soup makes a great winter dinner because it's packed with filling beans.

254 KCALS

TAKES 1 HOUR 25 MINUTES

● **SERVES 8**

2 tbsp sunflower oil
2 onions, chopped
1 tsp turmeric powder
1 tsp ground ginger
1 tbsp ground coriander
1 tbsp medium curry powder
1.25kg/2lb 12oz carrots, of which 1kg/2lb 4oz roughly sliced, rest coarsely grated
3 x 400g cans butter beans, drained and rinsed
1.2 litres/2 pints vegetable stock
400ml/14fl oz whole milk
snipped chives, to garnish (optional)

1 Put the oil and onions in the biggest pan or casserole you have and cook for 10 minutes to soften the onions. Stir in the spices and cook for 2 minutes, then add the sliced carrots with half the beans and the vegetable stock. Bring to a simmer, then cover and cook for 15–20 minutes until the carrots are tender.

2 Whizz the soup to a purée with a hand blender, or purée in batches in a blender or food processor. Tip the soup back into the pan (pour it through a sieve or a colander, if you like) and stir in the remaining beans and the grated carrot with 500ml/18fl oz hot water. Bring back to a simmer, then cover and cook gently for 10 minutes.

3 Stir in the milk and season to taste, then keep on a very gentle heat until needed. If you like, snip a few chives over and serve with crusty bread.

PER SERVING 254 kcals, protein 13g, carbs 36g, fat 6g, sat fat 2g, fibre 12g, sugar 18g, salt 1.8g

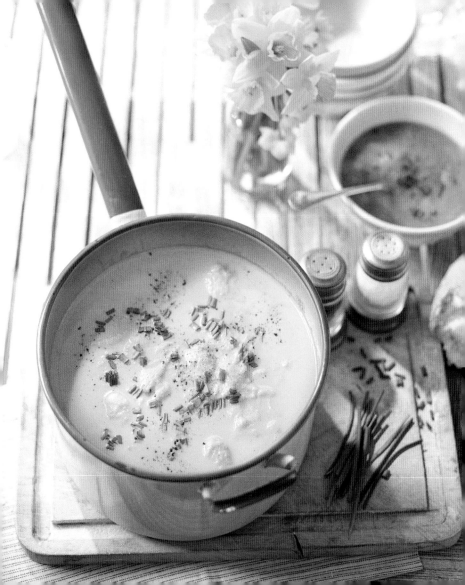

Carrot & sesame burgers

Burgers are a family staple, and these sesame-scented ones can be dressed up or down, depending on who likes what in your house.

284 KCALS

TAKES 50 MINUTES ● **MAKES 6**

750g/1lb 10oz carrots,
    peeled and grated
410g can chickpeas,
    drained and rinsed
1 small onion, roughly chopped
2 tbsp tahini paste, plus extra 1 tsp
    for sauce
1 tsp ground cumin
1 egg
3 tbsp olive oil
100g/4oz wholemeal breadcrumbs
zest of 1 lemon, plus 1 tsp juice
3 tbsp sesame seeds, toasted
150g pot natural yogurt

1 Put a third of the grated carrot in a food processor with the chickpeas, onion, tahini, cumin and egg. Whizz to a thick paste, then scrape into a bowl.
2 Heat 1 tablespoon of the oil in your largest frying pan, tip in the remaining carrot, then cook for 8–10 minutes, stirring until soft. Add the cooked carrot to the whizzed paste with the breadcrumbs, lemon zest and sesame seeds. Add seasoning, then mix together.
3 Divide the mixture into six, then using wet hands shape into burgers. Cover and chill until serving. Mix the yogurt with the extra tahini and the lemon juice. Chill.
4 Brush the burgers with the remaining oil. Fry or grill the burgers for 5 minutes on each side, until golden and crisp.
5 When the burgers are ready, serve in toasted buns with some of the lemony sesame yogurt, and some avocado, sliced onion, rocket and chilli sauce, if you like.

PER BURGER 284 kcals, protein 10g, carbs 27g, fat 16g, sat fat 3g, fibre 7g, sugar 12g, salt 0.5g

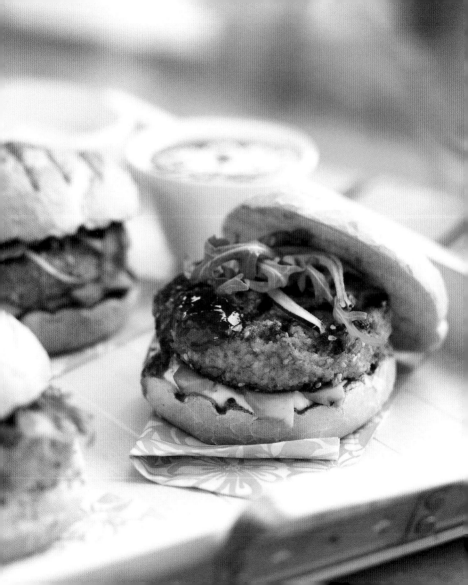

Prawn & pink-grapefruit noodle salad

Take a healthy Vietnamese approach to salads by using low-fat rice noodles with a sweet dressing and plenty of flavourful herbs.

228 KCALS

TAKES 25 MINUTES • SERVES 6

200g/7oz thin rice noodles
12 cherry tomatoes, halved
1 tbsp Thai fish sauce
juice 1 lime
2 tsp palm sugar or soft brown sugar
1 large red chilli, deseeded ½ diced,
　½ sliced
2 pink grapefruits, segmented
½ cucumber, peeled, deseeded and
　thinly sliced
2 carrots, cut into matchsticks
3 spring onions, thinly sliced
400g/14oz large cooked peeled prawns
large handful each mint and coriander,
　leaves picked

1 Put the noodles in a large bowl, breaking them up a little, and cover with boiling water from the kettle. Leave to soak for 10 minutes until tender. Drain, rinse under cold running water and leave the noodles to drain thoroughly.

2 In the same bowl, lightly squash the cherry tomatoes – we used the end of a rolling pin. Stir in the fish sauce, lime juice, sugar and diced chilli. Taste for the right balance of sweet, sour and spicy – adjust if necessary.

3 Toss through the noodles, then add all the remaining ingredients, except the sliced chilli. Season and give everything a good stir, then divide among six serving dishes and sprinkle over the sliced chilli.

PER SERVING 228 kcals, protein 13g, carbs 38g, fat 1g, sat fat none, fibre 2g, sugar 6g, salt 1.6g

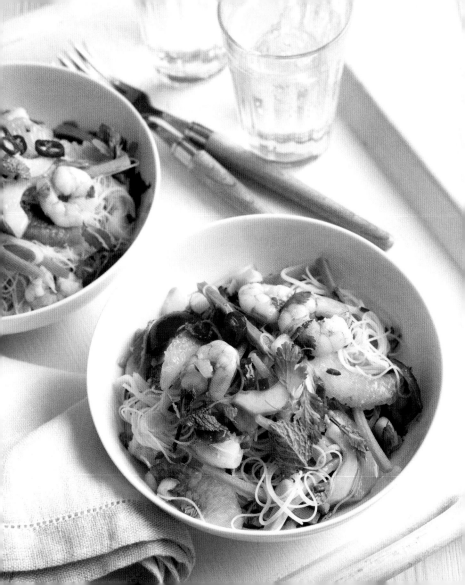

Grilled salmon tacos with chipotle-lime yogurt

Grill healthy fish with smoky chipotle spice then serve with cabbage salad, coriander and chilli in soft tortillas.

297 KCALS

TAKES 25 MINUTES ● COOK 10 MINUTES ● SERVES 4

1 tsp garlic salt
2 tbsp smoked paprika
good pinch sugar
500g/1lb 2oz salmon fillet
200g/7oz fat-free natural yogurt
1 tbsp chipotle paste or hot chilli sauce
juice 1 lime

TO SERVE

8 small soft flour tortillas, warmed
¼ small green cabbage, finely shredded
small bunch coriander, picked
    into sprigs
few pickled jalapeño chillies, sliced
lime wedges

1 Rub the garlic salt, paprika, sugar and some seasoning into the flesh of the salmon fillet. Heat grill to high.

2 Mix the yogurt, chipotle paste or hot sauce and lime juice together in a bowl with some seasoning, and set aside. Put the salmon on a baking sheet lined with foil and grill, skin-side down, for 7–8 minutes until cooked through. Remove from the grill and carefully peel off and discard the skin.

3 Flake the salmon into large chunks and serve with the warmed tortillas, chipotle-yogurt, shredded cabbage, coriander, jalapeños and lime wedges. Add a shake of hot sauce if you like it spicy.

PER SERVING 297 kcals, protein 33g, carbs 8g, fat 15g, sat fat 3g, fibre 5g, sugar 7g, salt 1.5g

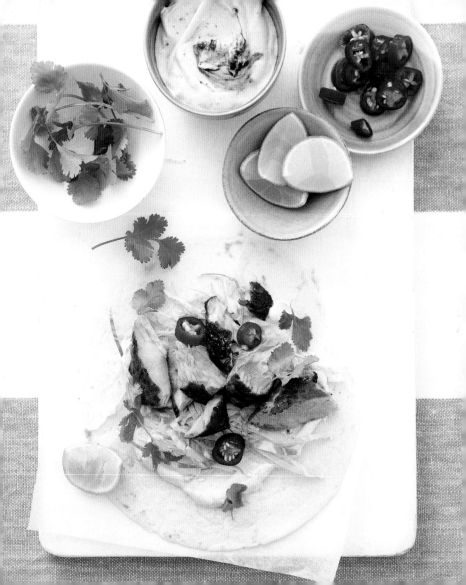

Creamy beetroot curry

This curry might sound unusual, but the earthy sweetness of beetroot works really well with Indian spices.

271 KCALS

TAKES 1 HOUR • **SERVES 4**

1 tbsp vegetable oil

2 onions, very finely chopped

2 tsp yellow mustard seeds

3 tbsp Madras curry paste

1kg/2lb 2oz (peeled weight) raw beetroot, peeled, halved and thickly sliced (wear gloves!)

1 green chilli, halved lengthways

400g can chopped tomatoes

3 tbsp ground almonds

4 tbsp low-fat natural yogurt, plus extra to garnish

1 Heat the oil in a large lidded pan, stir in the onions and cook for 8 minutes until soft. Tip in the mustard seeds and cook for 1 minute until toasted. Stir through the curry paste and sizzle for 3 minutes.

2 Mix the beetroot through the spicy onions, then add the chilli, tomatoes and 2 cans of water. Cover and simmer for 30 minutes until the beetroot is tender, stirring occasionally. Remove the lid, turn up the heat and cook until the sauce is thick.

3 Take off the heat, then stir through the almonds, yogurt and some seasoning. Serve topped with yogurt, with some basmati rice alongside, if you like.

PER SERVING 271 kcals, protein 11g, carbs 29g, fat 13g, sat fat 1g, fibre 7g, sugar 26g, salt 1g

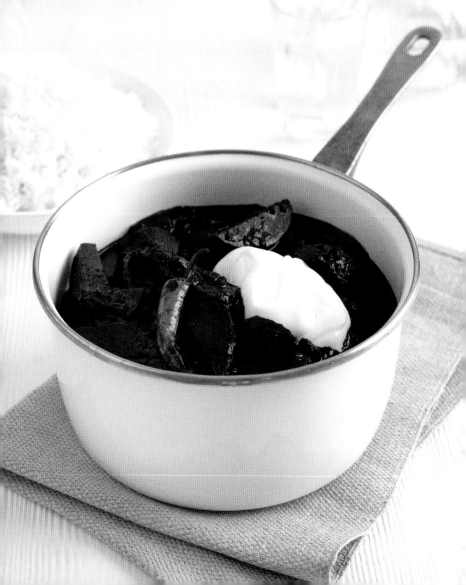

Chicken, ginger & green-bean hotpot

A light chicken casserole that makes a great Asian-inspired family one-pot.

215 KCALS

TAKES 30 MINUTES ● **SERVES 2**

½ tbsp vegetable oil

2cm/¾in piece ginger, cut into matchsticks

1 garlic clove, chopped

½ onion, thinly sliced

1 tbsp Thai fish sauce

½ tbsp light soft brown sugar

250g/9oz skinless chicken thigh fillets, trimmed of all fat and cut in half

125ml/4fl oz chicken stock

50g/2oz green beans, trimmed and cut into 2.5cm/1in lengths

1 tbsp coriander leaves, to garnish

1 Heat the oil in a pan over a medium-high heat. Add the ginger, garlic and onion, and stir-fry for about 5 minutes or until lightly golden. Add the fish sauce, sugar, chicken and stock. Cover and cook over a medium heat for 15 minutes.
2 For the final 3 minutes of cooking, add the green beans. Remove from the heat and stir through half of the coriander. Serve with steamed rice and the remaining coriander scattered over, if you like.

PER SERVING 215 kcals, protein 30g, carbs 9g, fat 7g, sat fat 1g, fibre 2g, sugar 7g, salt 2g

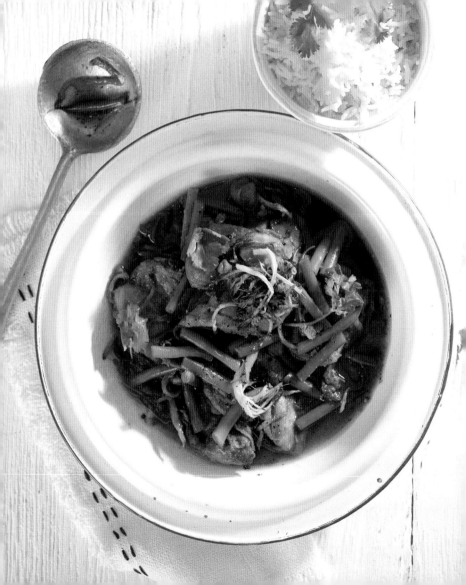

Low-fat moussaka

This summer-holiday favourite gets a healthy makeover by bulking up the mince with lentils and swapping to fat-free Greek yogurt.

289 KCALS

TAKES 55 MINUTES ● **SERVES 4**

200g/7oz frozen sliced peppers
3 garlic cloves, crushed
200g/7oz extra-lean beef mince
100g/4oz red split lentils
2 tsp dried oregano, plus extra for sprinkling
500ml carton passata
1 aubergine, sliced into 0.5cm/¼in rounds
4 tomatoes, sliced into 1cm/½in rounds
2 tsp olive oil
25g/1oz Parmesan, finely grated
170g pot fat-free Greek yogurt
freshly grated nutmeg

1 Cook the peppers gently in a large non-stick pan for about 5 minutes. Add the garlic and cook for 1 minute more, then add the beef, breaking it up with a fork, and cook until browned. Tip in the lentils, half the oregano, the passata and a splash of water. Simmer for 15–20 minutes until the lentils are tender, adding more water if you need to.

2 Meanwhile, heat the grill to medium-high. Arrange the aubergine and tomato slices on a non-stick baking sheet and brush with the oil. Sprinkle with the remaining oregano and some seasoning, then grill for 1–2 minutes each side until lightly charred; do this in batches if needed.

3 Mix half the Parmesan with the yogurt and some seasoning. Divide the beef mixture among four small ovenproof dishes; top with the sliced aubergine and tomato, then the yogurt mix, extra oregano, remaining Parmesan and nutmeg. Grill for 3–4 minutes until bubbling.

PER SERVING 289 kcals, protein 26g, carbs 31g, fat 8g, sat fat 3g, fibre 5g, sugar 12g, salt 1g

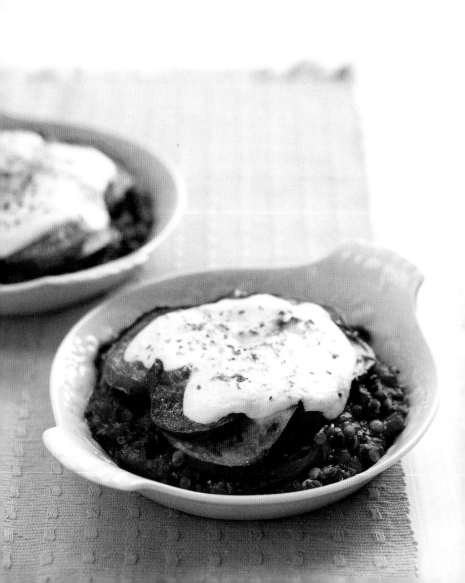

Faggots with onion gravy

Make a batch of these British classics, then you can freeze cooled portions in covered foil trays. Simply cook from frozen for 45–60 minutes at 200C/180C fan/gas 6.

TAKES 2 HOURS ● SERVES 8

oil, for greasing
170g pack sage and onion stuffing mix
500g pack diced pork shoulder
300g/10oz pig's liver
⅛ tsp ground mace
handful chopped parsley, to garnish

FOR THE GRAVY

2 onions, thinly sliced
1 tbsp sunflower oil
2 tsp sugar
1 tbsp red wine vinegar
3 tbsp plain flour
850ml/1½ pints beef stock

1 Heat oven to 160°C/140°C fan/gas 3. Lightly oil a very large roasting tin. Tip the stuffing mix into a large bowl, add 500ml/18fl oz boiling water, stir and set aside.

2 Pulse the pork in a food processor until finely chopped. Add the liver and pulse again. Add to the stuffing with the mace, 1 teaspoon salt and plenty of black pepper. Stir well. Shape the mixture into 24 large faggots and put in a roasting tin.

3 To make the gravy, fry the onions in the oil until starting to turn golden. Add the sugar and continue cooking, stirring frequently, until caramelised. Tip in the vinegar and allow to sizzle. Mix the flour with a couple of tablespoons water. Pour the stock into the onions, then add the flour paste and cook, stirring constantly, until smooth and starting to thicken. When it is thick, pour into the tin with the faggots, cover with foil and bake for 1 hour until cooked through. Serve sprinkled with parsley alongside the mash and veg, if you like.

PER SERVING 208 kcals, protein 26g, carbs 14g, fat 5g, sat fat 1g, fibre 2g, sugar 3g, salt 1.2g

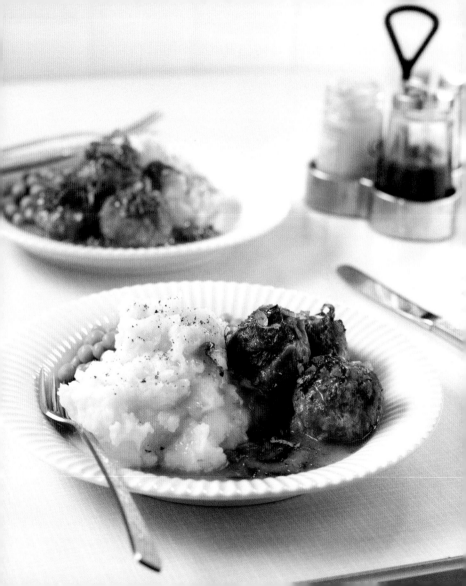

Moroccan roasted veg with tahini dressing

Tahini is a smooth paste made from sesame seeds – you might recognise its nutty flavour from good houmous.

272 KCALS

TAKES 45 MINUTES ● **SERVES 4**

2 courgettes, cut into chunks
3 red peppers, deseeded and
    cut into chunks
1 large aubergine,
    cut into chunks
8 spring onions, cut into
    2cm/¾in lengths
2 tbsp olive oil
2 tbsp harissa paste
2 tbsp tahini paste
juice 1 lemon
4 tbsp Greek yogurt
small bunch mint, roughly chopped

1 Heat oven to 200°C/180°C fan/gas 6. Spread the vegetables out on a baking sheet. Drizzle over the oil and harissa, season and toss well. Roast for 30 minutes or until cooked and beginning to caramelise.

2 Mix together the tahini, lemon juice, yogurt and 1–2 tablespoons water to make a dressing. Stir in half the mint.

3 Sprinkle the veg with the remaining mint and serve with the dressing, plus some couscous and warm pitta bread, if you like.

PER SERVING 272 kcals, protein 10g, carbs 15g, fat 19g, sat fat 5g, fibre 10g, sugar 14g, salt 0.2g

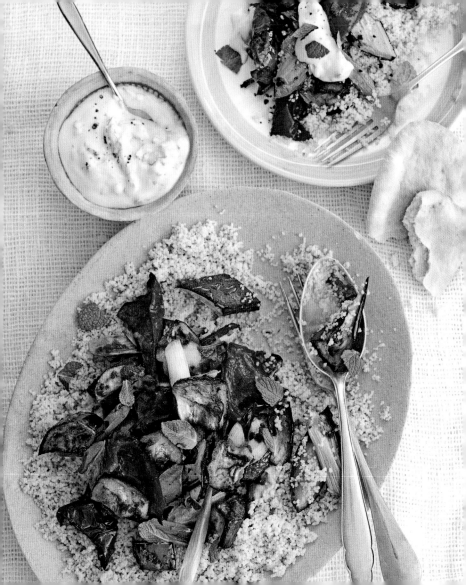

Sticky cod with celeriac & parsley mash

Ditch the Friday-night fish and chips, this lightly fried fillet is tasty and satisfying but a less heavy alternative.

259 KCALS

TAKES 35 MINUTES • SERVES 4

2 tbsp extra virgin olive oil
4 x 120g/4½oz pieces cod fillet
little plain flour, for dusting
2 garlic cloves, chopped
1 tsp crushed chilli flakes
3 tbsp sherry vinegar
1 tbsp light soft brown sugar
lemon wedges, to garnish

FOR THE MASH

1 large head celeriac (about 500g/1lb
   2oz), peeled and cubed
2 tbsp butter
big handful parsley, finely chopped

1 To make the mash, boil the celeriac in salted water for 10 minutes until soft. Drain, put back in the pan and steam-dry for a few minutes. Mash with the butter and seasoning, then stir in most of the parsley. Keep warm while you cook the fish.

2 Heat half the oil in a frying pan. Dust the fish in flour, season on both sides, and fry for about 4 minutes on each side. Remove to a plate. Add the remaining oil to the pan and cook the garlic and chilli for 2 minutes until golden. Add the vinegar, sugar and a little salt, then allow to bubble for 1–2 minutes. Return the fish to the pan to warm through.

3 Serve the fish on the mash, with the sauce from the pan poured over. Sprinkle with the remaining parsley and serve with lemon wedges.

PER SERVING 259 kcals, protein 25g, carbs 10g, fat 13g, sat fat 5g, fibre 7g, sugar 7g, salt 0.6g

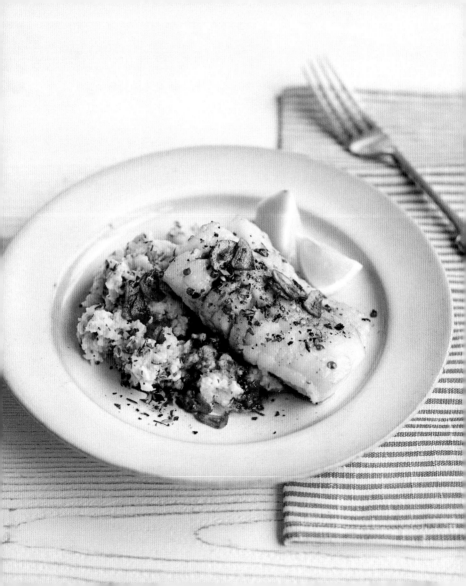

Chicken with mushrooms

A healthy chicken casserole with bacon, peas and mushrooms. You can use lower-fat breasts to make it even healthier, but thighs add extra flavour.

260 KCALS

TAKES 40 MINUTES ● **SERVES 4**

2 tbsp olive oil
500g/1lb 2oz boneless skinless
   chicken thighs
flour, for dusting
50g/2oz cubetti di pancetta (or
   smoked bacon lardons)
300g/10oz small button mushrooms
2 large shallots, chopped
250ml/9fl oz chicken stock
1 tbsp white wine vinegar
50g/2oz frozen peas
small handful parsley, finely chopped

1 Heat 1 tablespoon of the oil in a frying pan. Season and dust the chicken with flour and fry until brown on all sides. Remove and set aside. Fry the pancetta and mushrooms until softened, then remove.

2 Add the final tablespoon of oil and cook the shallots for 5 minutes. Add the stock and vinegar and bubble for 1–2 minutes. Return the chicken, pancetta and mushrooms to the pan and cook for 15 minutes. Add the peas and parsley and cook for 2 minutes more, then serve.

PER SERVING 260 kcals, protein 32g, carbs 3g, fat 13g, sat fat 3g, fibre 3g, sugar 1g, salt 0.9g

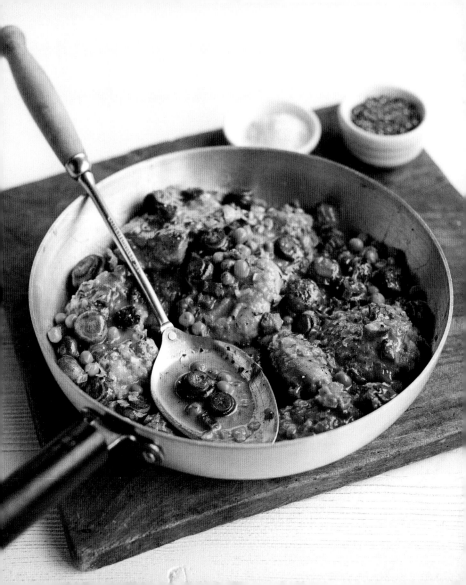

Minced beef & sweet potato stew

Thrifty lean mince makes a great base for a hearty, but healthy, family casserole.
Serve simply with seasonal greens.

368 KCALS

TAKES 20 MINUTES • SERVES 4

1 tbsp sunflower oil
1 large onion, chopped
1 large carrot, chopped
1 celery stick, sliced
500g/1lb 2oz lean beef mince
1 tbsp each tomato purée and
    mushroom ketchup
400g can chopped tomatoes
450g/1lb sweet potatoes, peeled and
    cut into large chunks
few thyme sprigs
1 bay leaf
handful parsley, chopped

1 Heat the oil in a large pan, add the onion, carrot and celery, and sweat for 10 minutes until soft. Add the beef and cook until it is browned all over.
2 Add the tomato purée and cook for a few minutes, then add the mushroom ketchup, tomatoes, sweet potatoes, herbs and a can full of water. Season well and bring to the boil.
3 Simmer for 40–45 minutes on a low heat until the sweet potatoes are tender, stirring a few times throughout to make sure they are cooking evenly.
4 Once cooked, remove the bay leaf, stir through the chopped parsley and serve with seasonal greens.

PER SERVING 368 kcals, protein 29g, carbs 35g, fat 13g, sat fat 5g, fibre 6g, sugar 17g, salt 0.6g

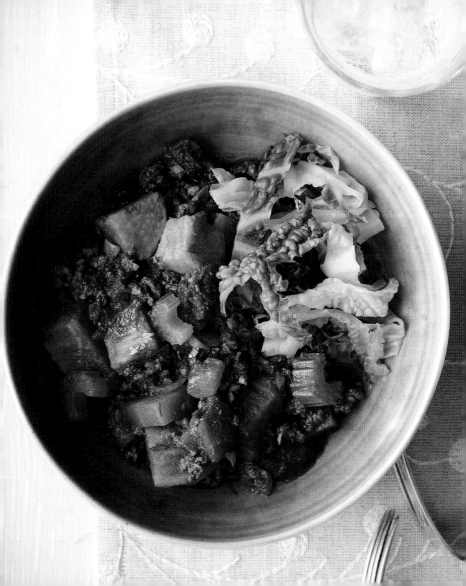

As-you-like-it tortilla

This tortilla uses leftovers as the main ingredient and matches them to a storecupboard flavour.

`343 KCALS`

TAKES 20 MINUTES ● SERVES 3

6 eggs

2 tsp pesto, or 1 tsp ready-made
    mustard or harissa paste, or
    2 tbsp chopped herb leaves

large handful leftovers such as
    chopped ham or chicken, tuna or
    flaked salmon

3 spring onions, finely chopped

125g/4½oz cooked pasta or 200g/7oz
    chopped cooked potato

handful veg such as frozen spinach
    or peas, drained canned corn,
    roasted peppers, fried courgettes
    or mushrooms

1½ tbsp vegetable oil

1 Beat the eggs with seasoning and your chosen background flavour, then add your leftovers. Stir in the spring onions and pasta or potatoes with your selected veg.

2 Heat the grill to high. Heat the oil in a medium non-stick frying pan and tip in the egg mixture. Cook gently for 10 minutes over a low heat until three-quarters set, then flash under the grill to set the top. Serve with a simple salad.

PER SERVING 343 kcals, protein 24g, carbs 16g, fat 20g, sat fat 6g, fibre 4g, sugar 2g, salt 2.1g

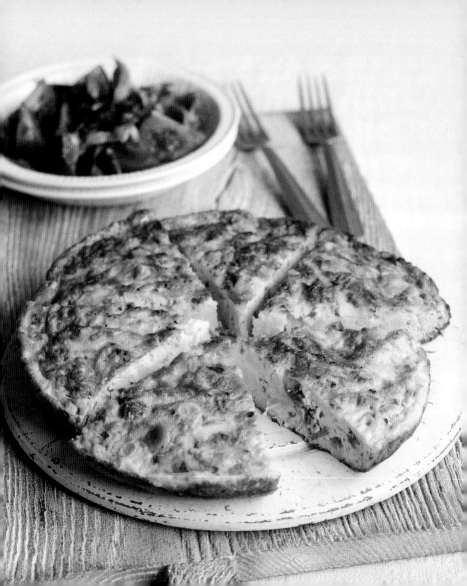

Oaty fish & prawn gratins

A creamy mash topped pie is packed with calories, but these crumb-topped, tomatoey versions are much healthier.

359 KCALS

TAKES 40 MINUTES • MAKES 2

340g bag baby leaf spinach,
   roughly chopped
400g can chopped tomatoes
   with garlic and herbs
225g/8oz sustainable white fish fillets,
   chopped into large chunks
small bunch basil, shredded
100g/4oz cooked peeled prawns
2 tbsp finely grated Parmesan
2 tbsp breadcrumbs
2 tbsp rolled oats
170g/6oz broccoli, boiled or steamed,
   to serve

1 Put the spinach in a large colander and pour over some boiling water. Once cool enough to handle, squeeze out any excess water, then season.
2 Tip the tomatoes into a frying pan with some seasoning and simmer for 5 minutes to thicken. Add the fish and heat for 1–2 minutes – it doesn't need to be fully cooked at this point. Stir in the basil.
3 Heat oven to 220°C/200°C fan/gas 7. Divide the prawns, spinach, fish and tomato sauce between two gratin dishes. Mix the Parmesan, breadcrumbs and oats together and sprinkle over the top. Bake for 20 minutes until golden and bubbling. Serve with cooked broccoli.

PER GRATIN 359 kcals, protein 48g, carbs 27g, fat 6g, sat fat 2g, fibre 8g, sugar 9g, salt 3.4g

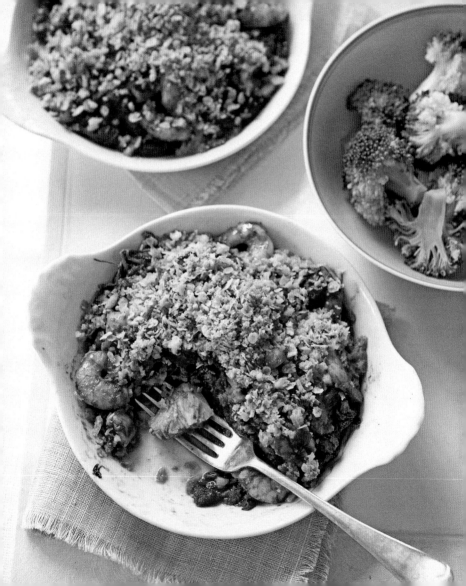

Farro salad with roasted carrots & feta

Farro is a wholegrain a bit like pearl barley, but instead of turning spongy when cooked it becomes chewy and nutty – perfect for salads.

370 KCALS

TAKES 35 MINUTES • SERVES 4

500g/1lb 2oz carrots, halved
    or quartered (baby carrots
    can stay whole)
2 red onions, quartered
1 tbsp extra virgin olive oil
200g/7oz farro or pearled spelt
100g/4oz baby leaf spinach
50g/2oz feta

FOR THE DRESSING

3 tbsp red wine vinegar
2 tbsp extra virgin olive oil
1 tbsp clear honey
2 garlic cloves, chopped
1 tsp each ground cumin and sweet
    smoked paprika
small handful parsley, finely chopped

1 Heat oven to 190°C/170°C fan/gas 5. Put the carrots and onions in a large roasting tin, drizzle with the oil and season well. Roast for 25 minutes.

2 While the vegetables are roasting, boil the farro or spelt according to the pack instructions. Drain and tip into a bowl. Mix the dressing ingredients with 1 tablespoon water and some seasoning, then stir half through the warm grains.

3 When the vegetables finish cooking, pour over the remaining dressing and mix well. Toss with the grains and spinach, then crumble over the feta.

PER SERVING 370 kcals, protein 12g, carbs 48g, fat 13g, sat fat 3g, fibre 9g, sugar 20g, salt 0.7g

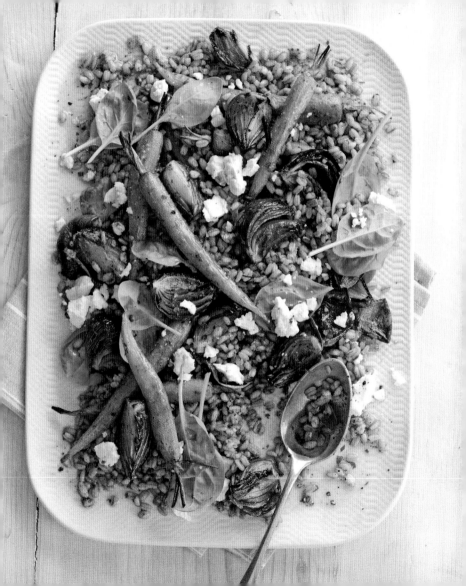

Crab & avocado tostadas

Canned crab and corn tortillas are great storecupboard standbys – keep them handy and supper is only 10 minutes away.

394 KCALS

TAKES 10 MINUTES ● MAKES 2

1 small red onion,
 sliced into thin rings
juice 2 limes, plus wedges
 to garnish
pinch caster sugar
170g can white crabmeat
 in brine, drained
2 spring onions, finely sliced
1 red chilli, deseeded and chopped
1 really ripe avocado, peeled, stoned
 and chopped
1 small garlic clove, crushed
2 corn tortillas
handful of mixed salad leaves

1 Put the onion in a bowl and cover with half the lime juice and a good pinch each of sugar and salt. Leave to soften while you get everything else ready.

2 Mix together the crab, spring onions and half the chilli. Season with black pepper and set aside.

3 Mash the avocado with the remaining lime juice, garlic and some seasoning. You can leave it quite chunky or mash it until smooth. Stir in the rest of the chilli.

4 Bend each tortilla in half and toast in a toaster for 1 minute. Flatten out again, put on two plates and top with the salad leaves, then the mashed avocado. Finish with the crabmeat and drained pickled onion. Serve with lime wedges for squeezing over.

PER TOSTADA 394 kcals, protein 22g, carbs 27g, fat 19g, sat fat 5g, fibre 6g, sugar 5g, salt 1.1g

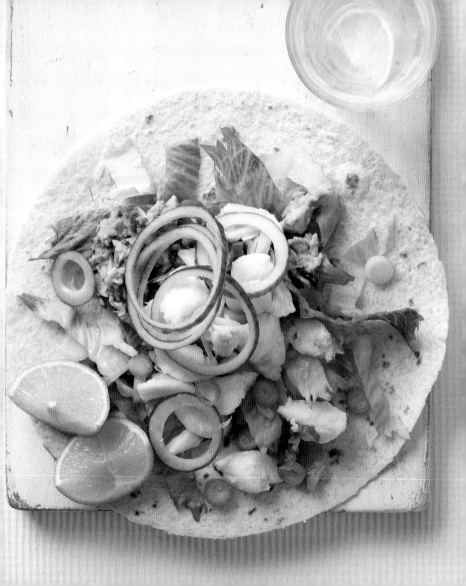

Chard, sweet potato & peanut stew

This vegan stew is great served with brown rice, and leftovers taste even better the next day.

398 KCALS

TAKES 1 HOUR • SERVES 4

2 tbsp sunflower oil
1 large onion, chopped
1 tsp cumin seeds
400g/14oz sweet potatoes, cut into medium chunks
½ tsp crushed chilli flakes
400g can chopped tomatoes
140g/5oz salted roasted peanuts
250g/9oz chard, leaves and stems, washed and roughly chopped

1 Heat a large pan with a lid. Add the oil, tip in the onion and fry until light golden. Stir in the cumin seeds until fragrant, then add the sweet potato, chilli flakes, tomatoes and 750ml/1¼ pints water. Stir, bring to the boil then simmer for 15 minutes.

2 Meanwhile, whizz the peanuts in a food processor until finely ground, but stop before you end up with peanut butter. Add them to the stew, then stir and season. Simmer for a further 15 minutes, stirring frequently.

3 Finally, stir in the chard. Return to the boil and simmer, covered, stirring occasionally, for 8–10 minutes or until the chard is cooked. Serve piping hot with plenty of freshly ground black pepper.

PER SERVING 398 kcals, protein 13g, carbs 33g, fat 25g, sat fat 4g, fibre 6g, sugar 12g, salt 0.93g

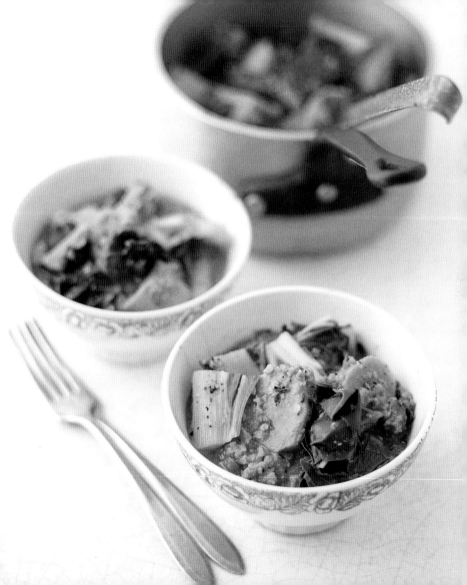

Pollack, beetroot & potato tray bake with lemony cream

Pollack is used here as it is one of the cheaper and most sustainable types of white fish, but you can substitute it for any firm white fish fillets you like.

336 KCALS

TAKES 55 MINUTES • SERVES 4

4 small potatoes, sliced

1 tbsp olive oil

2 tsp fennel seeds, lightly crushed

4 raw beetroot, peeled and cut
   into wedges

4 pollack fillets

zest ½ lemon

4 tbsp crème fraîche

small handful basil leaves,
   roughly torn

1 Heat oven to 200°C/180°C fan/gas 6. Put the potatoes in a large roasting tin and toss with the olive oil and fennel seeds. Season, arrange in a single layer, then bake for 20 minutes until softened and starting to crisp on the outside.

2 Turn the potatoes over and add the beetroot, season and return to the oven for 15 minutes. Remove the veg from the oven and sit the fish centrally on top of the veg. Season well and rub over a little oil from the tin. Return to the oven for 10 minutes more.

3 Meanwhile, in a small bowl, sprinkle the lemon zest over the crème fraîche with a good grind of black pepper. To serve, scatter the fish with basil and dollop with some of the lemony crème fraîche.

PER SERVING 336 kcals, protein 26g, carbs 31g, fat 12g, sat fat 6g, fibre 3g, sugar 4g, salt 0.4g

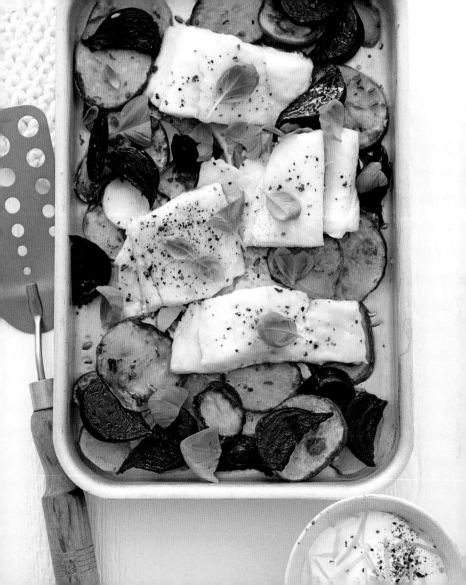

Quinoa stew with squash & pomegranate

This one-pot needs no accompaniments, so you can enjoy a filling supper for less than 320 calories!

318 KCALS

TAKES 55 MINUTES • SERVES 4

1 small butternut squash, deseeded
   and cubed
2 tbsp olive oil
1 large onion, thinly sliced
1 garlic clove, chopped
1 tbsp finely chopped ginger
1 tsp ras-el-hanout or Moroccan
   spice mix
200g/7oz quinoa
5 prunes, roughly chopped
juice 1 lemon
600ml/1 pint vegetable stock
seeds from 1 pomegranate and
   small handful mint leaves,
   to garnish

1 Heat oven to 200°C/180°C fan/gas 6. Put the squash on a baking sheet and toss with 1 tablespoon of the oil. Season well and roast for 30–35 minutes, or until soft.

2 Meanwhile, heat the remaining oil in a big pan. Add the onion, garlic and ginger, season and cook for 10 minutes. Add the spice mix and quinoa and cook for another couple of minutes. Add the prunes, lemon juice and stock, bring to the boil, then cover and simmer for 25 minutes.

3 When everything is tender, stir the squash through the stew. Spoon into bowls and scatter with pomegranate seeds and mint to serve.

PER SERVING 318 kcals, protein 11g, carbs 50g, fat 9g, sat fat 1g, fibre 6g, sugar 20g, salt 0.5g

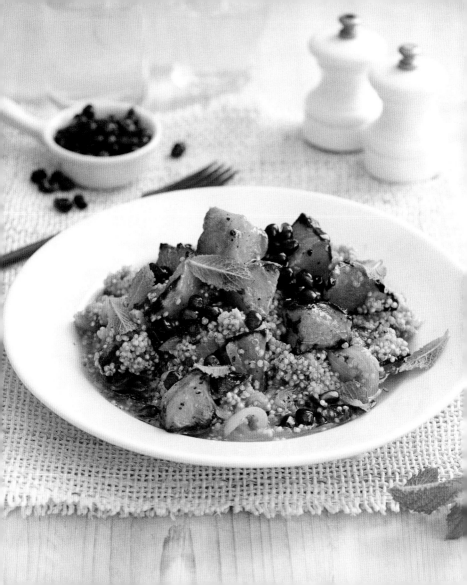

Spicy prawn pizzas

Butterflying prawns opens them out, which always seems to make the prawns go further! Make a cut along the prawn belly, open it out and press it down.

352 KCALS

TAKES 30 MINUTES, PLUS RISING
● **SERVES 4**

FOR THE DOUGH

250g pack white bread mix
2 tbsp extra virgin olive oil, plus extra
plain flour, for ducting

FOR THE SAUCE

200g can chopped plum tomatoes
1 tbsp tomato purée
1 garlic clove, crushed
pinch sugar (caster or granulated)

FOR THE TOPPING

3 tbsp each mascarpone and finely
    grated Parmesan
10 cherry tomatoes, halved
12 large raw peeled prawns, patted
    dry, deveined and butterflied
2 rosemary sprigs, needles
    roughly chopped
generous pinch chilli flakes
handful pitted green olives, halved
small drizzle extra virgin olive oil

1 Make the dough the day before. Put the bread mix in a large bowl, then tip in the oil with 150ml/¼ pint warm water. Stir to a soft dough and set aside for 5 minutes.
2 Knead the dough for 5 minutes on a floured surface until springy and smooth. Squish some extra oil around in a large food bag, then pop in the dough and tie the top, leaving room for the dough to grow. Leave to rise in the fridge.
3 To make the sauce, stir the ingredients together. When ready to cook, heat the oven as high as it will go. Dust a large baking sheet and work surface with flour. Split the dough in half. Roll into large slipper shapes, about 30cm/12in long, and lift them on to the baking sheet.
4 Spread the sauce over, then scatter with small dollops of mascarpone, the Parmesan, cherry tomatoes, prawns, rosemary, chilli flakes, olives, seasoning. and a little oil. Bake for 10–13 minutes until the base is crisp and the prawns are cooked through. Serve straight away.

PER SERVING 352 kcals, protein 19g, carbs 34g, fat 15g, sat fat 6g, fibre 3g, sugar 4g, salt 1.3g

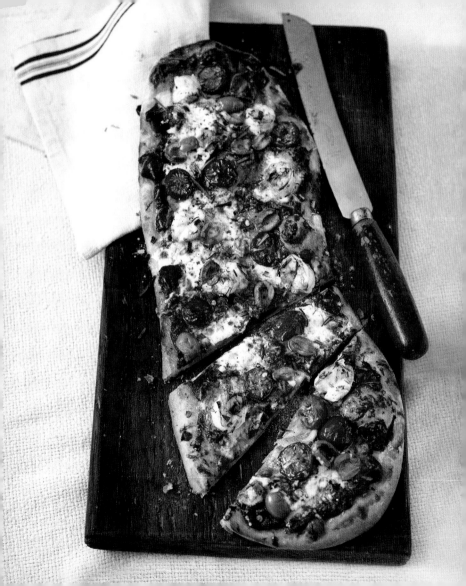

Oriental salmon & broccoli tray bake

Five ingredients are all you need to create this Asian-flavoured fish dish with healthy greens and lemon.

310 KCALS

TAKES 30 MINUTES • **SERVES 4**

4 skin-on salmon fillets
1 head broccoli, broken into florets
juice ½ lemon, other ½ quartered
small bunch spring onions, sliced
a little olive oil, to drizzle
2 tbsp light soy sauce

1 Heat oven to 180°C/160°C fan/gas 4. Put the salmon in a large roasting tin, leaving space between each fillet.
2 Wash and drain the broccoli and, while still a little wet, arrange in the tin around the fillets. Pour the lemon juice over everything, then add the lemon quarters.
3 Top with half the spring onions, drizzle with a little olive oil and put in the oven for 14 minutes. Remove from the oven, sprinkle everything with the soy sauce, then return to the oven for 4 minutes more until the salmon is cooked through. Sprinkle with the remaining spring onions just before serving.

PER SERVING 310 kcals, protein 35g, carbs 3g, fat 17g, sat fat 3g, fibre 4g, sugar 3g, salt 1.6g

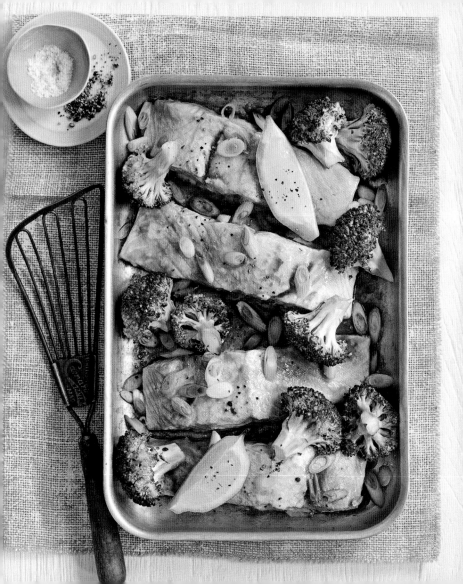

Harissa-aubergine kebabs with minty carrot salad

These North African-inspired kebabs are also great cooked on the barbecue come the warmer weather.

TAKES 25 MINUTES ● SERVES 2

2 tbsp harissa paste
2 tbsp red wine vinegar
1 aubergine, cut into 4cm/1½in cubes
2 carrots, finely shredded
1 small red onion, sliced
small handful mint, chopped,
    plus extra leaves to garnish
2 Middle Eastern flatbreads
2 heaped tbsp houmous
fat-free Greek yogurt, to serve

1 Mix the harissa and vinegar in a bowl. Remove half and reserve. Toss the aubergine in the remaining harissa sauce and season. Thread on to metal or soaked wooden skewers. Heat a griddle or grill until hot, then cook the kebabs until golden on all sides and cooked through.

2 Meanwhile, mix together the carrots, onion and chopped mint with some seasoning.

3 Top the flatbreads with the houmous, carrot salad and kebabs. Scatter over the extra mint leaves and serve with yogurt and a drizzle of the reserved harissa sauce.

PER SERVING 353 kcals, protein 13g, carbs 54g, fat 8g, sat fat 1g, fibre 13g, sugar 19g, salt 1.7g

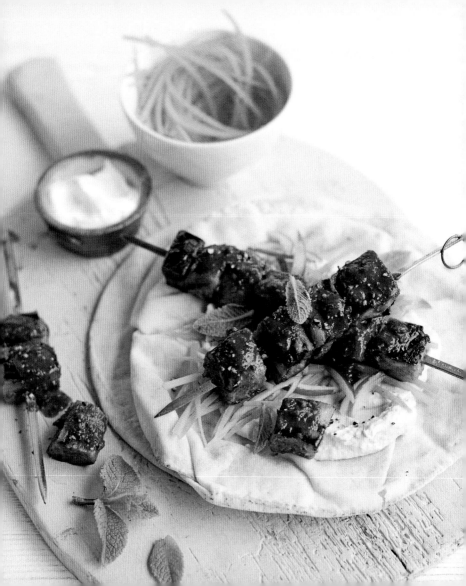

Turkey tortilla pie

Kids will absolutely love this tasty Tex-Mex twist on a shepherd's pie – especially the crisp cheesy topping!

369 KCALS

TAKES 30 MINUTES • SERVES 4

2 onions, finely chopped

1 tbsp olive oil, plus a little extra, if needed

2 tsp ground cumin

500g pack turkey mince

1½ tbsp chipotle paste

400g can chopped tomatoes

400g can kidney beans, drained and rinsed

198g can sweetcorn, drained and rinsed

2 soft corn tortillas, snipped into triangles

small handful grated Cheddar

2 spring onions, finely sliced

1 In a deep flameproof casserole dish, cook the onions in the oil until soft. Add the cumin and cook for 1 minute more. Stir in the mince and add a bit more oil, if needed. Turn up the heat and cook for 4–6 minutes until the mince is browned, stirring occasionally.

2 Stir in the chipotle paste, tomatoes and half a can of water, and simmer for 5 minutes. Mix in the beans and sweetcorn and cook for a few minutes more until thick, piping hot and the mince is cooked.

3 Heat the grill to medium-high. Take the pan off the heat and put the tortilla triangles randomly on top. Scatter over the cheese and grill for a few minutes until the topping is crisp, taking care that it doesn't burn. Sprinkle with the spring onions and serve.

PER SERVING 369 kcals, protein 42g, carbs 25g, fat 11g, sat fat 4g, fibre 6g, sugar 10g, salt 2.5g

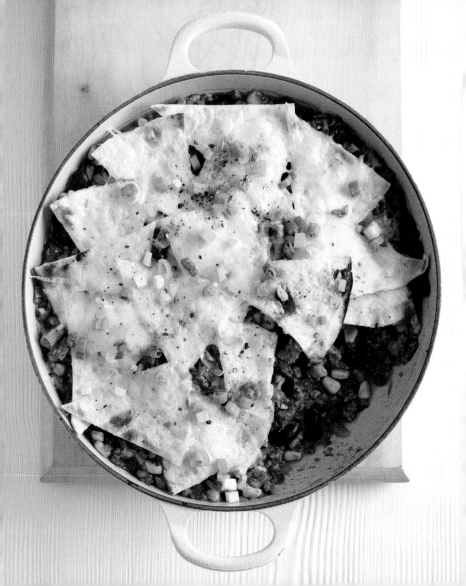

Fragrant fish tagine

Special enough for entertaining but light enough to fit in with your healthy-eating regime. Serve this with basmati rice, boiled with a little saffron, if you're really hungry.

282 KCALS

TAKES 1 HOUR ● SERVES 8

FOR THE CHERMOULA & FISH

2 tbsp olive oil
4 garlic cloves, roughly chopped
4 tsp ground cumin
2 tsp paprika
bunch coriander, chopped
juice and zest 1 lemon
8 x 100g/4oz skinless tilapia fillets

FOR THE TAGINE

2 tbsp olive oil
2 large onions, halved and thinly sliced
2 garlic cloves, sliced
2 tsp each ground cumin and paprika
3 x 400g cans chopped tomatoes
500ml/18fl oz fish stock
175g/6oz pimento-stuffed olives
4 green peppers, quartered, deseeded and sliced
500g bag baby new potatoes, halved lengthways

1 To make the chermoula, put the oil, garlic, cumin, paprika, three-quarters of the coriander and 1 teaspoon salt in a small bowl. Add the lemon juice, then blitz with a hand blender until smooth. Spoon half over the fish fillets and turn them over to coat both sides. Set aside to marinate.

2 Heat the oil for the tagine and fry the onions and garlic until softened and starting to colour, about 4–5 minutes. Add the cumin and paprika and cook for 2 minutes more. Add the tomatoes, stock, olives and lemon zest, stir in the remaining chermoula and simmer, uncovered, for 10 minutes.

3 Stir in the peppers and potatoes, cover and simmer for 15 minutes until the potatoes are tender.

4 Stir the remaining coriander into the tagine, then arrange the fish fillets on top, and simmer gently for 4–6 minutes until the fish is just cooked.

PER SERVING 282 kcals, protein 24g, carbs 24g, fat 11g, sat fat 2g, fibre 5g, sugar 7g, salt 2.76g

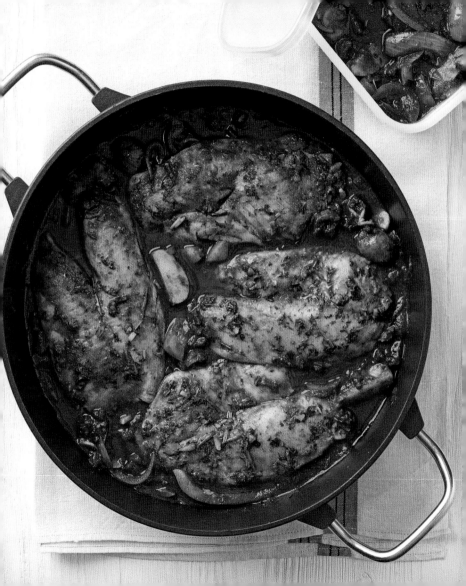

Bombay potato & spinach pies

These are ideal for a lunch with salad or as part of a buffet, but the quantities are easily halved if you just fancy making one.

386 KCALS

TAKES 1¼ HOURS • MAKES 2 (EACH SERVES 4)

FOR THE FILLING

1.25kg/2lb 12oz large waxy potatoes such as Charlotte, halved

2 onions, chopped

85g/3oz butter

1 tbsp each cumin seeds and black mustard seeds

2 tbsp finely chopped ginger

2 red chillies, halved, deseeded and sliced

3 tbsp korma curry paste

400g bag spinach leaves

4 tomatoes, chopped

small bunch coriander, chopped

FOR THE PASTRY

270g pack filo pastry (6 large sheets)

50g/2oz butter, melted

1 tsp black mustard seeds

1 Heat oven to 190°C/170°C fan/gas 5. Boil the potatoes for 15 minutes until tender. Fry the onions in the butter for a few minutes. Add the cumin and mustard seeds, ginger and chillies and fry until softened. Stir in the curry paste.

2 Cook the spinach in the microwave on High for 5 minutes. Drain, squeeze out as much liquid as you can, then chop. Drain the potatoes and crush into rough chunks with the spice mixture. Add the spinach, tomatoes and coriander, and season.

3 Unroll the pastry. Brush two 20cm loose-bottomed sandwich tins with butter. Brush a sheet of pastry with butter; lay it in the tin so it hangs over the side. Repeat with another sheet, so the two form a cross. Butter and fold a third sheet in half and lay it in the bottom to create a base. Repeat with the other tin and pastry.

4 Spoon in the filling and fold over the hanging pastry edges to enclose. Top with the remaining butter and the seeds. Bake for 35 minutes until golden and crisp.

PER SERVING 386 kcals, protein 9g, carbs 51g, fat 18g, sat fat 9g, fibre 5g, sugar 6g, salt 0.87g

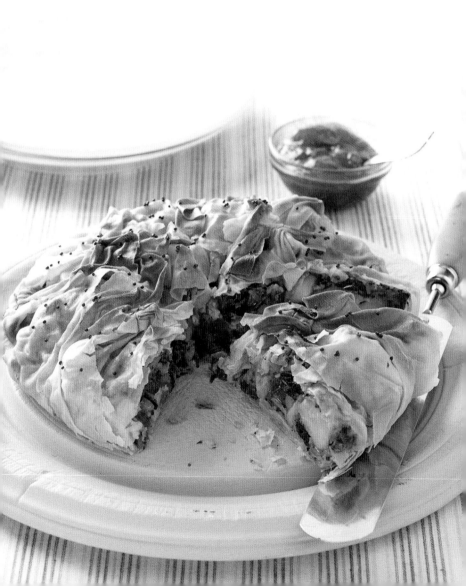

Chilli Marrakech

If your family loves spicy, aromatic dishes, this will instantly become a favourite. It uses lean lamb mince, although beef works well too. Serve with couscous or basmati rice.

357 KCALS

TAKES 1½ HOURS • SERVES 10

1½ tbsp cumin seeds

1 tbsp olive oil

3 onions, halved and thinly sliced

3 x 400g packs lean lamb mince

2 tbsp finely chopped ginger

4 garlic cloves, finely chopped

2 x 400g cans chopped tomatoes

1 tbsp each paprika and
    ground cinnamon

1½ tbsp ground coriander

3 tbsp harissa paste

3 red peppers, deseeded and
    cut into large chunks

2 x 400g cans chickpeas,
    drained and rinsed

2 x 20g packs coriander, most
    chopped, a few leaves left whole

500ml/18fl oz beef or lamb stock,
    made with 2 cubes

1 Heat your largest non-stick wok or pan, tip in the cumin seeds and toast for a few seconds then remove and set aside. Add the oil to the pan and fry the onions for 5 minutes until starting to colour. Add the mince, ginger and garlic, and cook, breaking up the mince with your wooden spoon, until the meat is no longer pink. Drain any excess liquid or fat from the pan.

2 Stir in the tomatoes, toasted cumin seeds, remaining spices and harissa. Add the peppers, chickpeas, three-quarters of the chopped coriander and the stock. Cover and cook for 40 minutes, stirring occasionally, until the sauce is slightly thickened.

3 Remove from the heat, then stir in the remaining chopped coriander. Serve scattered with the reserved coriander leaves.

PER SERVING 357 kcals, protein 28g, carbs 17g, fat 19g, sat fat 8g, fibre 5g, sugar 7g, salt 1.2g

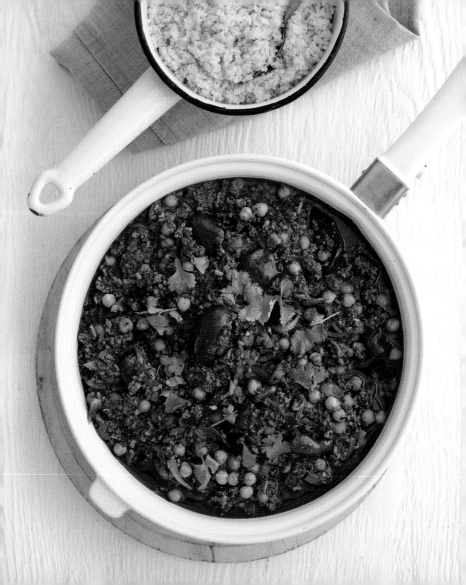

Smoked trout, beetroot & horseradish flatbreads

Crisp wraps work really well as a light pizza-style base. Try this Scandi topping first, then experiment with your other favourites.

327 KCALS

TAKES 18 MINUTES ● MAKES 4

4 flatbreads
olive oil, for brushing
2 tbsp horseradish sauce
2 tbsp crème fraîche
small bunch dill, ½ chopped,
    ½ picked into small fronds
squeeze of lemon juice, plus a
    pinch of zest
3 cooked beetroots (not in vinegar),
    very thinly sliced
4 smoked trout fillets, broken
    into large flakes

1 Heat oven to 220°C/200°C fan/gas 7. Brush the flatbreads with olive oil. Put on a large baking sheet and pop in the oven for about 8 minutes until crisp round the edges.

2 Meanwhile, mix the horseradish, crème fraîche, chopped dill, lemon juice and zest and some seasoning. Add a few drops of water to loosen the mixture to a drizzling consistency.

3 Top each flatbread with some beetroot slices and smoked trout. Drizzle over the horseradish sauce, sprinkle with dill fronds and serve with salad, if you like.

PER FLATBREAD 327 kcals, protein 21g, carbs 42g, fat 10g, sat fat 4g, fibre 3g, sugar 5g, salt 2.1g

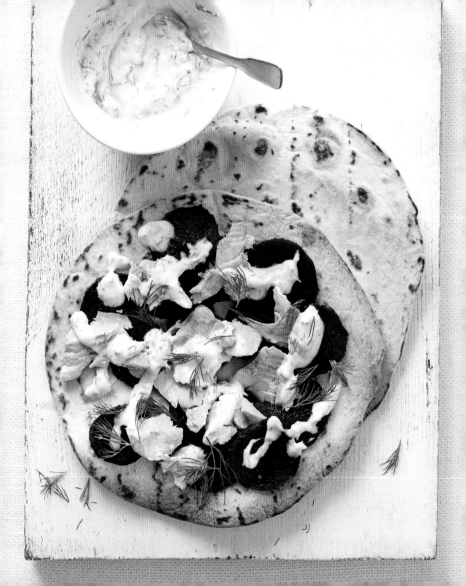

Chicken tikka with spiced rice

Our delicious version of this favourite is healthier than the average takeaway. By boiling the rice with spices we've packed in the flavour and cut the calorie content.

342 KCALS

TAKES 30 MINUTES, PLUS MARINATING • SERVES 4

4 boneless skinless chicken breasts

150g pot low-fat natural yogurt

50g/2oz tikka curry paste

100g/4oz cucumber, diced

1 tbsp roughly chopped mint leaves

1 red onion, cut into thin wedges

140g/5oz easy cook long grain rice

1 tbsp medium curry powder

50g/2oz frozen peas

1 small red pepper, deseeded and diced

1 Slash each chicken breast deeply with a knife three to four times on one side. Put in a bowl and add 50g/2oz of the yogurt and the tikka paste. Mix well, cover and marinate in the fridge for 30 minutes. Make the raita by stirring the cucumber and most of the mint into the rest of the yogurt. Season, cover and chill.

2 Heat oven to 240°C/220°C fan/gas 9. Scatter the onion over a foil-lined baking sheet. Remove the chicken from the marinade, shake off any excess and put on top of the onion. Cook for 20 minutes.

3 Meanwhile, tip the rice, curry powder, peas and pepper into a pan of boiling water and simmer for 10 minutes or until the rice is just tender. Drain well and divide the rice among four plates. Add the chicken, roasted onion and remaining mint. Serve with the cucumber raita.

PER SERVING 342 kcals, protein 37g, carbs 38g, fat 5g, sat fat 1g, fibre 4g, sugar 7g, salt 0.7g

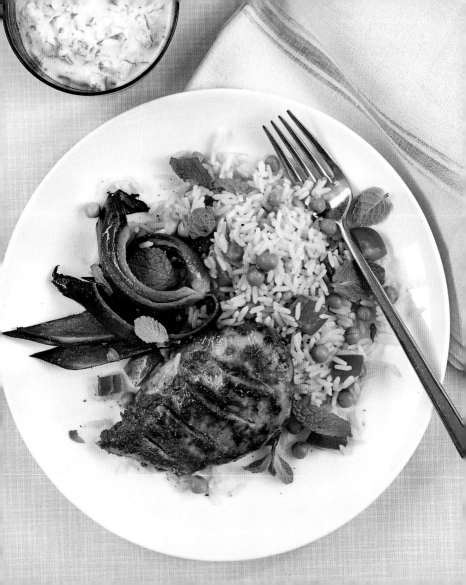

Chicken katsu

Crunchy breadcrumbed chicken and Japanese curry sauce — what more could you want for dinner? Great served with rice and soya beans with finely sliced red chilli.

319 KCALS

TAKES 40 MINUTES • SERVES 4

4 boneless skinless chicken breasts

1 egg, beaten

8 tbsp finely crushed cornflakes or Panko crumbs

2 garlic cloves, crushed

1–2 tbsp korma curry paste

1 tbsp light soy sauce

4 tbsp tomato ketchup

2 tbsp honey

2 tbsp cornflour

1 Heat oven to 200°C/180°C fan/gas 6. Dip the chicken in the egg, then coat in the cornflakes or crumbs. Space out the chicken breasts on a non-stick baking sheet and cook for 15–20 minutes or until cooked through.

2 Put the remaining ingredients in a pan. Pour in 500ml/18fl oz water and heat, stirring, until boiling and thickened. Cover and leave to simmer for 5 minutes.

3 Spoon some sauce on to four plates, slice the chicken breasts and put on top.

PER SERVING 319 kcals, protein 34g, carbs 36g, fat 5g, sat fat 1g, fibre none, sugar 13g, salt 2g

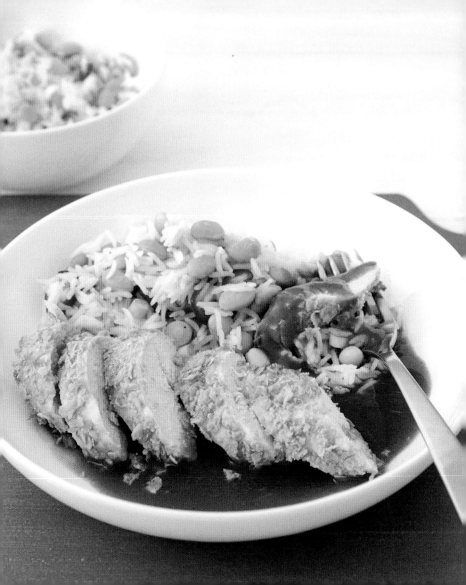

Courgette & ricotta tart

Topping this tart with ricotta and green veg makes the dish much lighter than you expect. Serve with a green salad and you'll only add a few more calories to supper.

341 KCALS

TAKES 50 MINUTES ● **SERVES 6**

2 tbsp olive oil
2 courgettes, thinly sliced
250g tub ricotta
2 eggs, beaten with a fork
small handful basil leaves, shredded
pinch grated nutmeg
1 tbsp grated Parmesan
   (or vegetarian alternative)
1 garlic clove, crushed
320g pack ready-rolled puff pastry
flour, for dusting

1 Heat oven to 200°C/180°C fan/gas 6. Heat half the oil in a frying pan. Cook the courgettes until golden around the edges, then remove from the pan and set aside. Mix together the ricotta, eggs, most of the basil, the nutmeg, Parmesan and garlic in a bowl.
2 Unroll the pastry on a lightly floured surface – roll it out lightly to make it a little thinner. Lay it on a baking sheet.
3 Spread the pastry with the ricotta mix, leaving a small border around the edge, then press the courgette slices into the ricotta. Bring the pastry sides up over the edge of the filling and pinch so that none seeps out the sides.
4 Bake for 30 minutes until the tart is puffed up and golden. Serve warm, scattered with the remaining basil.

PER SLICE 341 kcals, protein 11g, carbs 21g, fat 24g, sat fat 11g, fibre 1g, sugar 2g, salt 0.6g

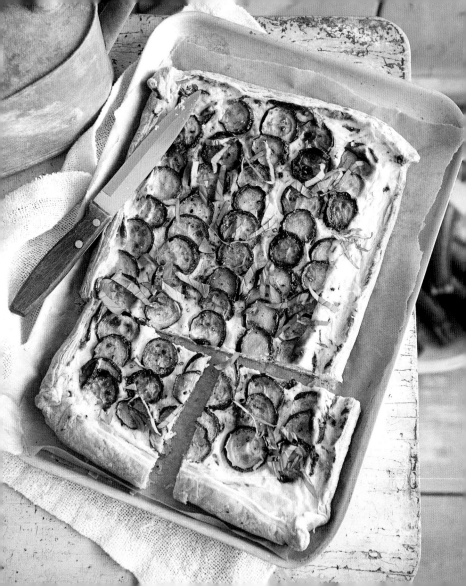

Easy chicken pies

A mash topped pie is much lower in calories than one made with buttery pastry, but no less satisfying on a cold night.

462 KCALS

TAKES 45 MINUTES • MAKES 4

1 onion, sliced

400g pack boneless skinless chicken thighs, cut into chunks

1 tbsp vegetable oil

150ml/¼ pint chicken stock

325g can sweetcorn, drained and rinsed

6 tbsp crème fraîche

handful parsley or basil leaves, chopped or torn

750g/1lb 10oz potatoes, cut into chunks

1 Heat oven to 180°C/160°C fan/gas 4. Fry the onion and chicken in the oil for 5–10 minutes until the onion is soft and the chicken golden. Pour over the stock, bring to the boil, then simmer for 20 minutes until the chicken is cooked. Stir in the corn, then add 3 tablespoons of the crème fraîche and the herbs.

2 Meanwhile, boil the potatoes until soft. Drain and mash with the remaining crème fraîche. Spoon the chicken mix into four pie dishes and top with mash. Put on a baking sheet, then grill until the potato is golden.

PER PIE 462 kcals, protein 29g, carbs 53g, fat 16g, sat fat 7g, fibre 4g, sugar 10g, salt 0.93g

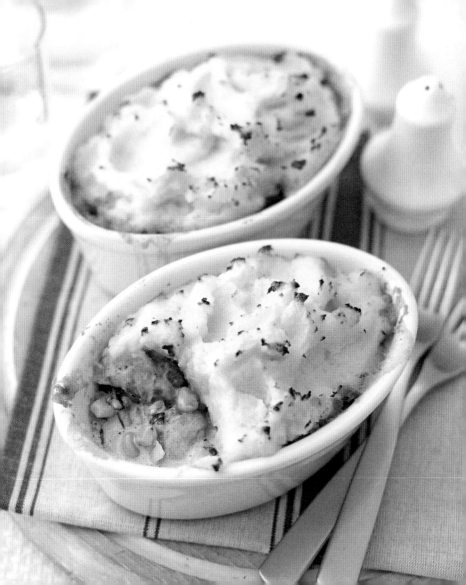

Fried fish & tomato curry

Use a sustainable white fish like pollack in this southern Indian style coconut and tomato curry.

432 KCALS

TAKES 35 MINUTES ● **SERVES 4**

2 tbsp vegetable oil, plus 2 tsp

2 onions, thinly sliced

8 large vine tomatoes, roughly chopped

4 garlic cloves

thumb-sized piece ginger, roughly
    chopped

3 tbsp madras curry paste

165ml can coconut milk

large handful coriander leaves, finely
    chopped, plus extra sprigs to garnish

500g/1lb 2oz firm white, skinless
    fish fillets

6 tbsp seasoned flour

1 Heat 2 teaspoons of the oil in a large frying pan. Tip in the onions and a pinch of salt. Cook until soft and golden.

2 Meanwhile, blitz the tomatoes, garlic and ginger in a food processor to a smooth purée. Add the curry paste to the onions and fry for 3 minutes more. Stir in the tomato mix and simmer for 10 minutes until thickened. Add the coconut milk and chopped coriander. Simmer again to thicken.

3 Dust the fish fillets in some seasoned flour. Heat the remaining oil in a non-stick frying pan. Cook the fillets, in batches, over a high heat for 1 minute or so on each side, until they begin to brown. Carefully place the fish in the tomato mixture and simmer until just cooked through. Scatter over the coriander sprigs and serve with rice, if you like.

PER SERVING 432 kcals, protein 30g, carbs 33g, fat 19g, sat fat 7g, fibre 5g, sugar 9g, salt 0.8g

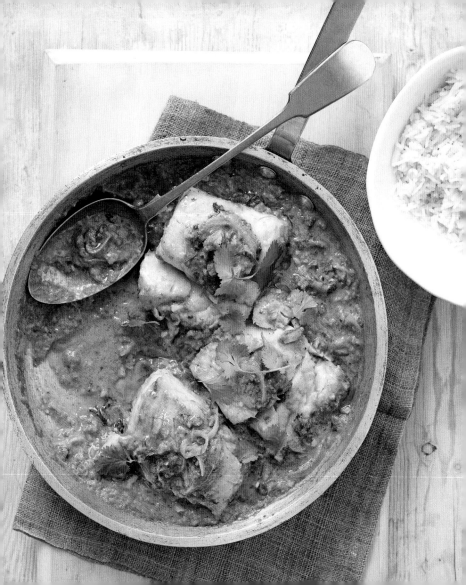

Cottage pie cakes

Lighter than a proper cottage pie but with all of the satisfaction – serve with low-sugar and salt baked beans.

426 KCALS

TAKES 35 MINUTES, PLUS CHILLING
● **MAKES 6**

400g/14oz pack lean beef mince
1 beef stock cube
50g/2oz plain flour
2 tbsp Worcestershire sauce
140g/5oz frozen peas
450g/1lb leftover mashed potatoes
2 eggs, beaten
85g/3oz panko or dried breadcrumbs
vegetable oil, for frying

1 Heat a large frying pan until hot. Dry-fry the mince until browned, breaking it up with a fork. Crumble in the stock cube and 1 tablespoon of the flour and mix well. Add the Worcestershire sauce and peas, and mix well to combine.

2 Tip the mince mixture into a bowl and cool a little, before stirring in the mash and shaping into six cakes. Dust the cakes in the remaining flour, then dip them into the egg, then the crumbs. Chill for at least 10 minutes, longer if you have time.

3 Heat the oil in a large pan. Fry the cakes for 3–4 minutes each side, until golden brown. Drain on kitchen paper. Season with a little salt and serve.

PER CAKE 426 kcals, protein 23g, carbs 31g, fat 25g, sat fat 7g, fibre 3g, sugar 2g, salt 1.22g

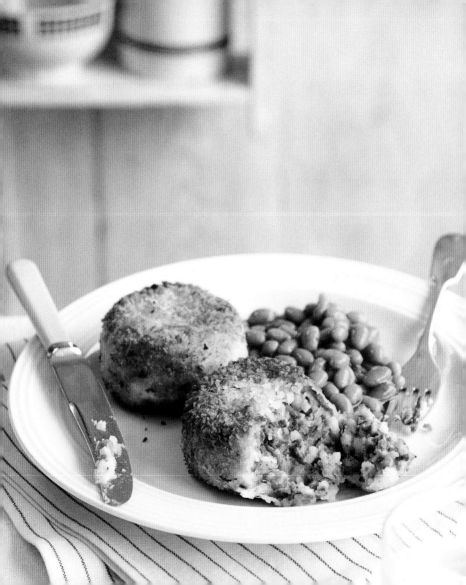

Spicy chicken, mango & jalapeño salad

This no-cook summer salad is packed with flavours and different textures, making it a really satisfying supper.

481 KCALS

TAKES 15 MINUTES • **SERVES 4**

250g pack cherry tomatoes,
  sliced or quartered
2 tbsp finely chopped jalapeños
small handful coriander leaves,
  roughly chopped
juice 1 lime, plus 4 halves to garnish
1 small red onion, finely chopped
1 tbsp extra virgin olive oil
4 cooked chicken breasts, torn into
  bite-sized shreds
2 Little Gem lettuces, torn into bite-
  sized pieces
1 red pepper, deseeded
  and sliced
1 ripe mango, stoned, peeled
  and diced
handful tortilla chips, broken,
  to sprinkle

1 Put the cherry tomatoes, jalapeños, coriander, lime juice, onion and oil in a large bowl with some seasoning.
2 Pop the remaining ingredients, except the tortilla chips, on top of the dressing. Gently mix the salad together to coat.
3 Sprinkle the tortilla chips over the top and serve immediately with lime halves.

PER SERVING 481 kcals, protein 22g, carbs 37g, fat 27g, sat fat 6g, fibre 6g, sugar 15g, salt 1.5g

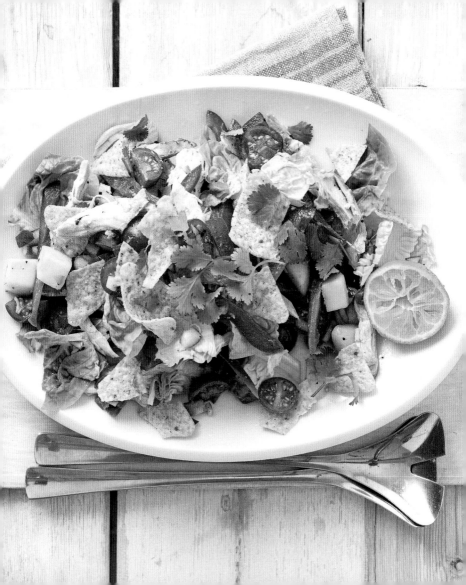

Healthier risotto primavera

Comfort food of the highest order, but we've made it much healthier without losing any flavour.

475 KCALS

TAKES 1¼ HOURS • SERVES 4

2 tbsp olive oil

350g/12oz asparagus, sliced into shorter lengths

1 bunch spring onions, sliced

175g/6oz frozen peas

250g/9oz shelled frozen broad beans

2 tbsp each shredded basil and snipped chives

1 tbsp finely chopped mint leaves

zest of 1 lemon

4 shallots, finely chopped

3 plump garlic cloves, finely chopped

300g/10oz risotto rice

150ml/¼ pint dry white wine

1.7 litres/3 pints hot vegetable bouillon

25g/1oz Parmesan, grated

25g/1oz rocket leaves

1 Heat half the oil in a frying pan. Tip in the asparagus and fry until browned. Stir in the spring onions and cook for 1–2 minutes. Remove; set aside. Boil the peas and beans for 3 minutes, then drain. Mix the herbs and lemon zest together.

2 Fry the shallots and garlic in the remaining oil in a big frying pan until soft. Stir in the rice for 2 minutes. As it starts to sizzle, pour in the wine and stir until absorbed. Start to stir in the hot stock, 1½ ladlefuls at a time, so it simmers and is absorbed after each addition. Keep stirring the whole time. After 20 minutes the rice should be soft with a bit of chew in the middle. Season.

3 Take off the heat. Pour over a ladleful of the remaining stock, scatter over the vegetables, half the herb mix and half the cheese. Cover and rest for 3–4 minutes.

4 Gently stir everything together, ladle into four dishes and top with the rocket, remaining herbs and cheese.

PER SERVING 475 kcals, protein 19g, carbs 71g, fat 10g, sat fat 3g, fibre 10g, sugar 5g, salt 0.3g

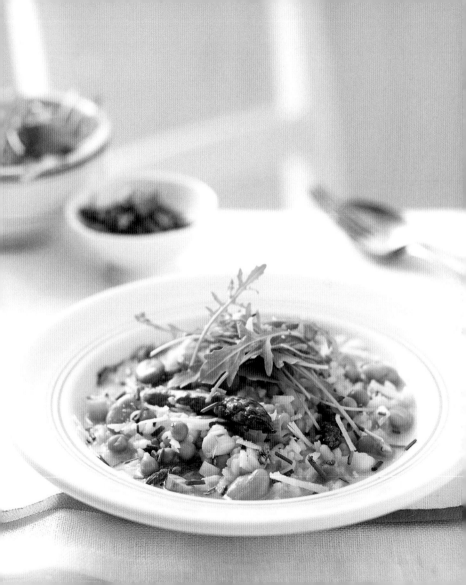

Greek beans with seared lamb

Lamb is a traditional topping for these Greek beans, but they'd also taste great with sliced chicken breast or pan-fried fish.

437 KCALS

TAKES 35 MINUTES ● **SERVES 4**

500g/1lb 2oz lamb fillet
1½ tbsp olive oil
3 garlic cloves, crushed
1 large onion, chopped
2 tbsp tomato purée
small bunch dill, most chopped, a few
    fronds left whole
1 tbsp red wine vinegar
500ml/18fl oz chicken stock
2 x 400g cans gigante or butter
    beans, drained and rinsed
2 tbsp crumbled feta

1 Rub the lamb with ½ tablespoon of the oil and a third of the crushed garlic. Season well and set aside to marinate while you prepare the beans, or for up to 2 hours if you have time.

2 Heat the remaining oil in a pan. Add the onion and remaining garlic, and season. Fry for 8 minutes until soft. Add the tomato purée, chopped dill, vinegar, stock and beans, season and simmer for 15 minutes or until most of the liquid has evaporated.

3 Meanwhile, heat a frying pan until hot. Sear the lamb on all sides, for about 5 minutes in total. Rest, covered with foil, for 5 minutes, then thickly slice. Serve the lamb with the beans, scattered with feta and the remaining dill sprigs.

PER SERVING 437 kcals, protein 34g, carbs 22g, fat 24g, sat fat 9g, fibre 8g, sugar 6g, salt 0.8g

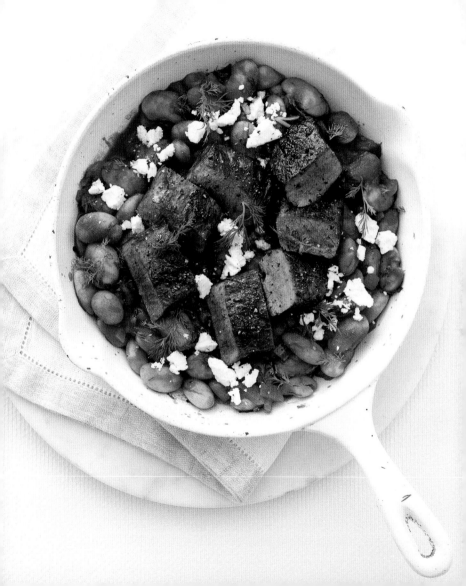

Spiced bulgar pilaf with fish

A pilaf is normally made with rice, but bulgar wheat is nutty and nutritious, so why not make a change?

416 KCALS

TAKES 45 MINUTES ● SERVES 4

1 tbsp olive oil
2 onions, finely sliced
3 carrots, grated
2 tsp cumin seeds
2 tbsp harissa paste
200g/7oz bulgar wheat
6 dried apricots, chopped
700ml/1¼ pints weak chicken stock
   (we used 1 stock cube)
200g/7oz baby leaf spinach
4 firm white fish fillets
4 thin lemon slices

1 Heat the oil in a lidded flameproof casserole dish. Tip in the onions and cook for 10 minutes until soft and golden. Add the carrots and cumin and cook for 2 minutes more. Stir through the harissa, bulgar and apricots, pour over the stock and bring to the boil. Cover and simmer for 7 minutes.

2 Add the spinach and stir through until just wilted. Arrange the fish fillets on top, pop a slice of lemon on each and season. Replace the lid and cook for 8 minutes, keeping it over a low-ish heat.

3 Turn the heat to low and cook for 7–8 minutes more until the fish is cooked through and the bulgar is tender. Season with freshly ground black pepper and serve.

PER SERVING 416 kcals, protein 37g, carbs 52g, fat 6g, sat fat 1g, fibre 7g, sugar 15g, salt 1g

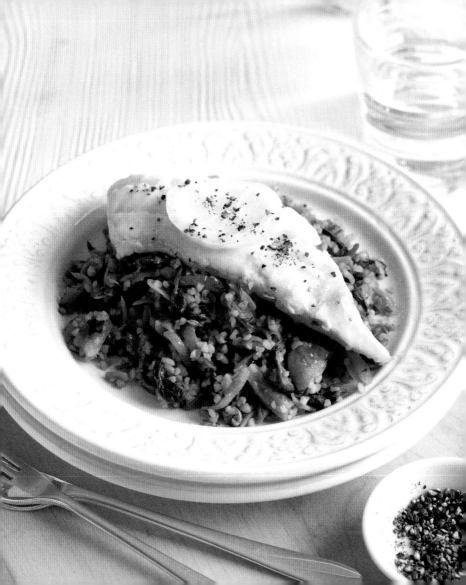

Tuna-sweetcorn cakes

When you haven't had time to hit the shops you might find yourself reaching for the takeaway menus – but stop! This supper can be rustled up from your storecupboard.

467 KCALS

TAKES 40 MINUTES, PLUS CHILLING
- **MAKES 4**

450g/1lb potatoes, quartered
2 tbsp mayonnaise, plus extra
    to serve
2 x 185g cans tuna, drained
198g can sweetcorn, drained
    and rinsed
small bunch chives, snipped, or
    1 tsp dried parsley
2 eggs, beaten
100g/4oz dried breadcrumbs
sunflower oil, for frying

1 Cook the potatoes in boiling salted water until really tender. Drain and allow to steam-dry in a colander. Tip into a bowl, season and mash. Stir in the mayonnaise, tuna, sweetcorn and chives or parsley. Shape into four cakes and chill until cold and firm.

2 Dip each cake into the egg, letting the excess drip off, then coat in the breadcrumbs. Chill for 15 minutes.

3 Heat a little of the oil in a pan and gently fry the cakes for 2–3 minutes on each side until golden. You may need to do this in batches – keep the cooked cakes warm in a low oven. Serve with extra mayonnaise and salad leaves, if you like.

PER CAKE 467 kcals, protein 27g, carbs 42g, fat 22g, sat fat 3g, fibre 3g, sugar 4g, salt 1.3g

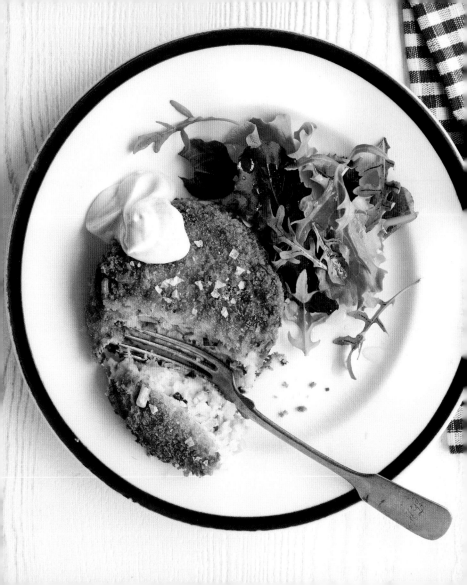

Jerk pork & pineapple skewers with black beans & rice

Spice up your low-cal supper with some Caribbean flavours – these skewers are great with chicken, too.

451 KCALS

TAKES 20 MINUTES ● MAKES 4

400g/14oz pork fillet,
    cut into 4cm/1½in chunks
2 tbsp jerk or Creole seasoning
1 tsp ground allspice
1 tbsp hot chilli sauce, plus extra to
    garnish (optional)
3 limes, zest and juice 1, other
    2 cut into wedges to serve
½ small pineapple, peeled, cored
    and cut into 4cm/1½in chunks
1 tbsp vegetable oil
200g/7oz basmati rice
400g can black beans,
    drained and rinsed

1 Mix together the pork, jerk or Creole seasoning, allspice, chilli sauce, if using, lime zest and juice and some seasoning. Thread the pork and pineapple on to metal skewers (or pre-soaked wooden skewers) and brush with the oil.

2 Cook the rice according to the pack instructions. Drain well, then put it back in the pan with the beans, stir and keep warm.

3 Meanwhile, heat a griddle pan until very hot. Cook the skewers for 3 minutes on each side until nicely charred and the pork is cooked through. Serve the skewers with the beans and rice, some extra chilli sauce, if you like, and lime wedges for squeezing over.

PER SKEWER 451 kcals, protein 30g, carbs 57g, fat 10g, sat fat 3g, fibre 6g, sugar 7g, salt 0.2g

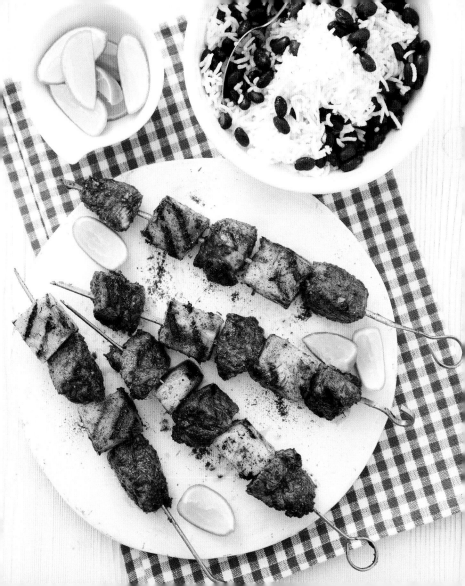

Pasta with ham & minty pea pesto

Ready-made pesto can be high in fat and calories, but by making your own you can vary the ingredients and keep it healthier.

487 KCALS

TAKES 22 MINUTES ● SERVES 4

400g/14oz pasta shapes

400g/14oz frozen peas, defrosted

½ bunch mint, leaves picked

50g/2oz grated Parmesan or pecorino, plus extra to taste (optional)

100g/4oz half-fat crème fraîche

175g/6oz thinly sliced smoked ham, shredded

1 Cook the pasta according to the pack instructions, adding half the peas for the final 1 minute of cooking. Drain, reserving some of the cooking water.

2 Meanwhile, blitz the rest of the peas, the mint leaves, half the Parmesan or pecorino and the crème fraîche until smooth, then season. When the pasta is cooked, tip it back into the pan on the heat and spoon in the pea cream, ham and the remaining cheese. Stir to coat the pasta evenly, adding the reserved water if it is too thick. Serve immediately, with extra Parmesan or pecorino, if you like.

PER SERVING 487 kcals, protein 30g, carbs 65g, fat 12g, sat fat 6g, fibre 7g, sugar 5g, salt 1.3g

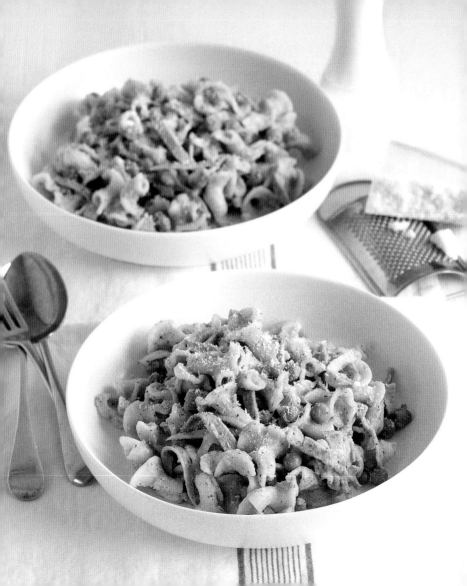

Miso-prawn skewers with veggie-rice salad

Seafood skewers and a veg-packed Japanese rice salad, all for less than 500 calories.

410 KCALS

TAKES 40 MINUTES • SERVES 4

200g/7oz brown basmati rice
175g/6oz mangetout
200g/7oz frozen soya beans
1½ tbsp sesame oil
4 spring onions, finely sliced
large handful coriander leaves,
  roughly chopped
1 green chilli, finely diced

FOR THE SKEWERS
400g/14oz large raw peeled prawns
3 tbsp sweet miso paste (find this in
  store with the Japanese ingredients)
2 tsp light soy sauce
2 tsp Japanese rice vinegar
2 tsp light soft brown sugar

1 Put the brown rice in a pan with lots of cold water. Bring to the boil and simmer for 20–25 minutes or until tender. Meanwhile, soak wooden skewers in some cold water (to prevent them burning). Add the mangetout and soya beans to the rice for the final 5 minutes of cooking. Rinse under cold water, draining thoroughly.

2 Toss the rice and veg with the sesame oil and mix in a large bowl with the spring onions, coriander, chilli and seasoning.

3 Preheat the grill to high. Put the skewer ingredients in a bowl with a few grinds of black pepper. Give everything a good stir, making sure the prawns are well coated. Thread the prawns on to the skewers and lay on a baking sheet. Grill for a couple of minutes on each side until the prawns are cooked through. Serve with the rice salad and drizzle over any of the cooking juices.

PER SERVING 410 kcals, protein 32g, carbs 47g, fat 10g, sat fat 2g, fibre 7g, sugar 8g, salt 1.5g

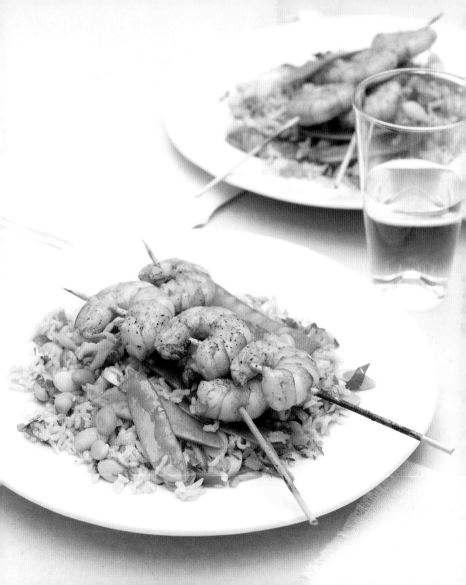

Turkey-chilli jacket potatoes

This healthy turkey chilli is also good on top of brown rice or baked sweet potatoes, or stuffed into peppers and cooked in the oven.

410 KCALS

TAKES 55 MINUTES (CHILLI ONLY)

- **SERVES 4**

4 large baking potatoes
1 tbsp olive oil
1 onion, chopped
1 garlic clove, crushed
300g/10oz turkey mince
1 tbsp each smoked paprika and
    ground cumin
1 tbsp cider vinegar
1 tbsp light soft brown sugar
350ml/12fl oz passata
reduced-fat Cheddar, grated, and
    chopped spring onions, to garnish

1 Heat oven to 200°C/180°C fan/gas 6. Use a fork to prick the potatoes all over. Rub with a little of the oil and bake for 45 minutes until tender.

2 Meanwhile, make the chilli. Heat the remaining oil in a large frying pan over a medium heat. Add the onion, garlic and some seasoning, and cook for 5 minutes until soft. Add the turkey mince and season again, then increase the heat and break up the mince with the back of a spoon. When the mince is cooked through, add the spices, vinegar, sugar and passata. Reduce to a simmer and cook for 10 minutes or until the liquid has reduced.

3 Cut a cross in the top of each potato and spoon in the chilli. Serve each potato sprinkled with the grated cheese and spring onions.

PER SERVING 410 kcals, protein 30g, carbs 61g, fat 5g, sat fat 1g, fibre 7g, sugar 13g, salt 0.1g

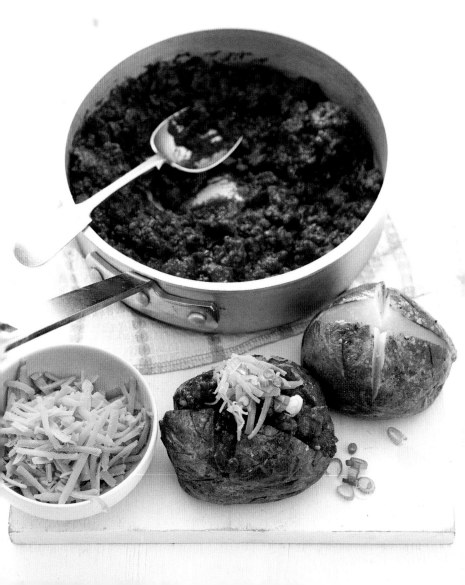

Chicken, butter bean & pepper stew

Swap half the chicken thighs for low-fat sausages if you want to mix this stew up a bit.

422 KCALS

TAKES 1 HOUR 5 MINUTES ● SERVES 4

1 tbsp olive oil
1 large onion, chopped
2 celery sticks, chopped
1 yellow and 1 red pepper,
    deseeded and diced
1 garlic clove, crushed
2 tbsp paprika
400g can chopped tomatoes
150ml/¼ pint chicken stock
2 x 400g cans butter beans, drained
    and rinsed
8 boneless skinless chicken thighs

1 Heat oven to 180°C/160°C fan/gas 4. Heat the oil in a large flameproof casserole dish. Add the onion, celery and peppers and fry for 5 minutes. Add the garlic and paprika, and cook for a further 3 minutes.

2 Stir in the tomatoes, stock and butter beans, and season well. Bring to the boil, then nestle the chicken thighs into the sauce. Cover with a tight-fitting lid and put in the oven for 45 minutes.

PER SERVING 422 kcals, protein 44g, carbs 27g, fat 15g, sat fat 4g, fibre 9g, sugar 12g, salt 1.6g

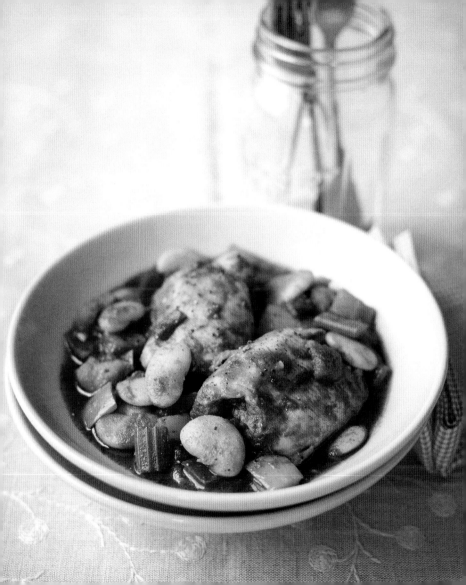

Teriyaki chicken meatballs with rice & greens

Try a healthy family supper with a difference with these chicken patties served in a sweet Japanese sauce.

481 KCALS

TAKES 25 MINUTES • SERVES 4

2 shallots
1 carrot, cut into chunks
500g/1lb 2oz boneless skinless
   chicken breasts or thighs,
   cut into chunks
zest and juice 1 lemon
a little oil
200g/7oz basmati rice
200g/7oz spring greens, chopped
100ml/3½fl oz mirin
3 tbsp dark soy sauce
3 tbsp caster sugar

1 Heat oven to 200°C/180°C fan/gas 6. Pulse the shallots and carrot in a food processor until finely chopped. Add the chicken, lemon zest and some seasoning, and pulse again until mixed. Using oiled hands, shape into small meatballs. Put the meatballs on a baking sheet lined with baking parchment and bake for 10 minutes until browned and cooked through.

2 Meanwhile, boil the rice according to the pack instructions, adding the spring greens for the final 4 minutes. Drain well.

3 Put the mirin, soy, lemon juice and sugar in a pan and bring to the boil, then reduce the heat and simmer until saucy. Remove from the heat, add the meatballs to the pan and roll them around in the sauce. Divide the rice and greens among four plates or bowls and spoon over the meatballs.

PER SERVING 481 kcals, protein 36g, carbs 70g, fat 2g, sat fat 1g, fibre 3g, sugar 28g, salt 2.3g

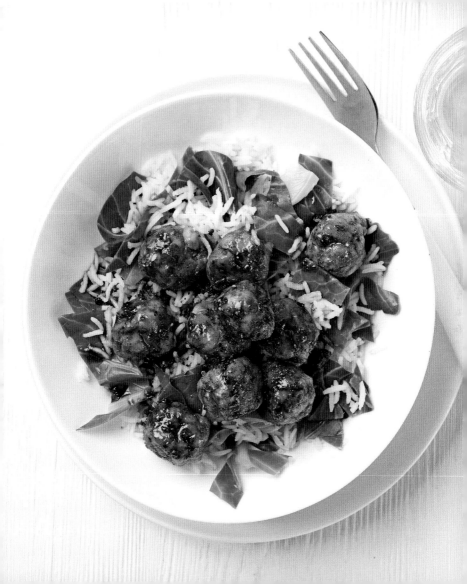

Spanish seafood pasta

Have this deliciously different pasta dish on the table in only 20 minutes from start to finish.

429 KCALS

TAKES 20 MINUTES • SERVES 4

350g/12oz short pasta shapes
  (we used orzo)
1 chicken stock cube, crumbled
1 tsp turmeric powder or a large pinch
  of saffron threads
85g/3oz chorizo, diced
200g pack cooked mixed seafood
2 roasted red peppers from a jar, sliced
100g/4oz frozen peas
2 tbsp chopped parsley

1 Cook the pasta in a pan according to the pack instructions, adding the stock cube and half the turmeric or saffron.
2 About 7 minutes before the pasta is cooked, tip the chorizo into a frying pan and cook over a medium heat for 5 minutes until slightly crisp. Tip out some of the fat, then add the remaining turmeric or saffron, the seafood, peppers and peas.
3 Drain the pasta, reserving some of the stock. Tip the pasta back into the pan, add the chorizo-and-seafood mixture and a splash of the reserved stock and heat through. Stir in most of the parsley.
4 Serve in warm bowls, with the remaining parsley sprinkled on top.

PER SERVING 429 kcals, protein 24g, carbs 67g, fat 7g, sat fat 3g, fibre 5g, sugar 3g, salt 1.2g

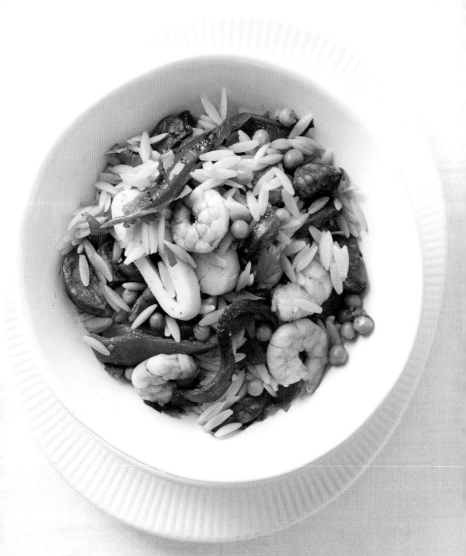

Summer-fruit compote

Combining berries and sweet plums makes for a really nutritious breakfast – a couple of dollops of low-fat yogurt will finish it off nicely.

98 KCALS

TAKES 15 MINUTES ● **SERVES 4**

4 large plums, stoned and
   cut into wedges
200g punnet blueberries
zest and juice 1 orange
25g/1oz light soft brown sugar
150g punnet raspberries

1 Cook the plums and blueberries in a small pan with the orange zest and juice, sugar and 4 tablespoons water until slightly softened but not mushy. Gently stir in the raspberries and cook for 1 minute more.

2 Remove from the heat and allow to cool to room temperature. Serve with low-fat yogurt, if you like.

PER SERVING 98 kcals, protein 2g, carbs 22g, fat none, sat fat none, fibre 4g, sugar 21g, salt none

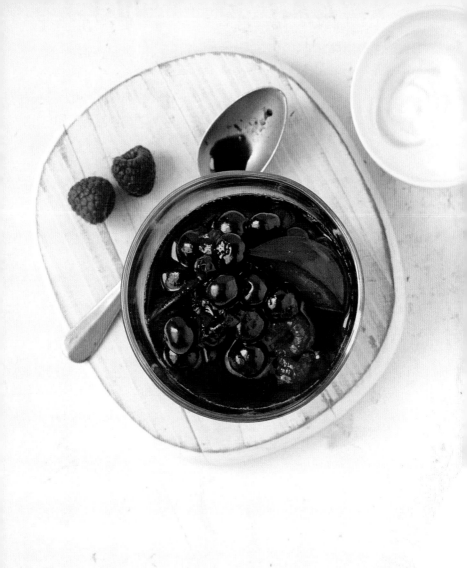

Grapefruit, orange & apricot salad

If you want to make this all year round, swap the fresh apricots for canned ones, but make sure they are in natural juice, not sugary syrup.

83 KCALS

TAKES 10 MINUTES • SERVES 4

2 grapefruits
4 oranges
4 apricots, stoned and sliced
1 tbsp clear honey

1 First segment the grapefruits and oranges. One by one, cut a little horizontal slice from the top and bottom of each fruit so that they can sit flat on a board. Using a small, sharp knife, cut off the peel and pith in downward strokes, following the curve of the fruit. Work your way round until all the peel is removed.
2 Hold the fruit over a bowl to catch the juice and then cut free each segment by carefully slicing between the membranes to release it. Put the segments into the bowl of juice and gently stir in the apricots and honey, and serve.

PER SERVING 83 kcals, protein 2g, carbs 18g, fat none, sat fat none, fibre 4g, sugar 18g, salt none

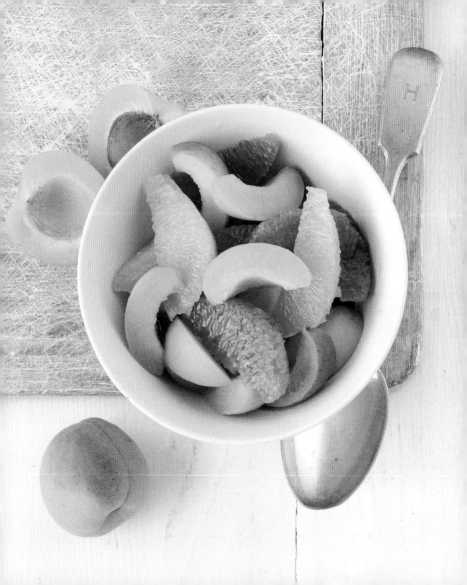

Apricot & raspberry tart

Filo pastry is naturally very low in fat, unlike most pastries, so it is a great ingredient to use if you're dieting.

150 KCALS

TAKES 40 MINUTES ● CUTS INTO 4 SLICES

3 large sheets filo pastry (or 6 small)
2 tbsp butter, melted
3 tbsp apricot conserve
6 ripe apricots, stoned and
    roughly sliced
85g/3oz raspberries
2 tsp caster sugar

1 Let the filo come to room temperature for about 10 minutes before use. Put a baking sheet into the oven and heat oven to 200°C/180°C fan/gas 6.
2 Brush each large sheet of filo with melted butter, layer them on top of each other, then fold each one in half so you have a smaller rectangle six layers thick. If using small sheets just stack them on top of each other. Fold in the edges of the pastry base to make a 2cm/¾in border, then spread the apricot conserve inside the border. Carefully slide the pastry base on to the hot baking sheet and bake for 5 minutes.
3 Remove from the oven, arrange the apricots over the tart and brush with any leftover melted butter. Bake for another 10 minutes, then scatter on the raspberries and sprinkle with sugar. Bake for a final 10 minutes until the pastry is golden brown and crisp.

PER SLICE 150 kcals, protein 2g, carbs 22g, fat 7g, sat fat 4g, fibre 2g, sugar 18g, salt 0.33g

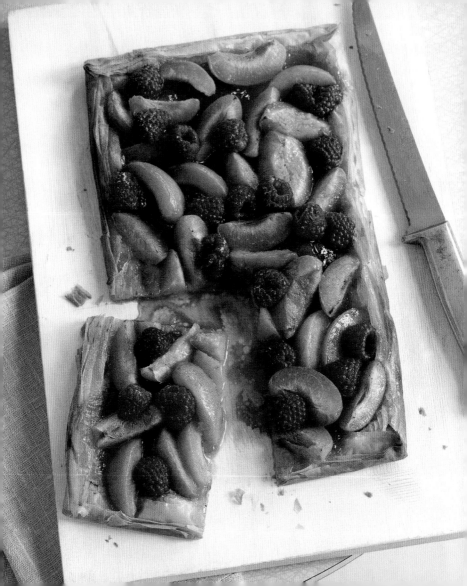

Healthier Victoria sandwich

Make it citrussy by stirring the finely grated zest of 1 orange or lemon into the cake mix, or spoon the mix into paper cases to make cupcakes or fairy cakes.

263 KCALS

TAKES 45 MINUTES • **CUTS INTO 8 SLICES**

2 tbsp rapeseed oil, plus extra for the tins
175g/6oz self-raising flour
1½ tsp baking powder
140g/5oz golden caster sugar
25g/1oz ground almonds
2 eggs
175g/6oz natural yogurt
2–3 drops vanilla extract
25g/1oz butter, melted
4 tbsp raspberry conserve
½ tsp icing sugar, to dust

1 Heat oven to 180°C/160°C fan/gas 4. Lightly oil two 18cm sandwich tins and line the bases with baking parchment. Tip the flour, baking powder, sugar and ground almonds into a large mixing bowl, then make a well in the centre. Beat the eggs in a bowl, then stir in the yogurt and vanilla. Pour this mixture, along with the melted butter and oil, into the dry mixture and stir until well combined.

2 Divide the mixture evenly between the tins and level the tops. Bake both cakes, side by side, for 20 minutes until risen and beginning to come away slightly from the edges of the tins.

3 Remove the cakes from the oven and loosen the sides with a round-bladed knife. Let the cakes cool in the tins, then turn them out. Peel off the lining paper and sit the cakes on a wire rack. Cool.

4 Put one of the cakes on a plate and spread over the conserve. Put the other cake on top and sift over the icing sugar.

PER SLICE 263 kcals, protein 5.6g, carbs 39g, fat 9.3g, sat fat 2.8g, fibre 1.3g, sugar 24.1g, salt 0.6g

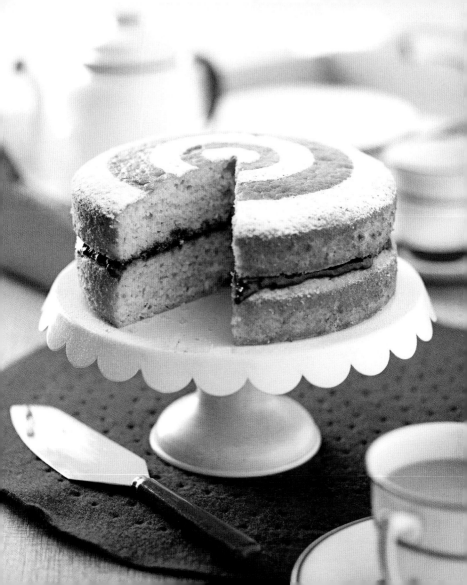

Guilt-free bread & butter pudding

We've worked wonders with this naughty pud, so that you can diet and still enjoy it.

312 KCALS

TAKES 55 MINUTES, PLUS SOAKING AND INFUSING • SERVES 4

50g/2oz dried apricots, chopped
25g/1oz raisins
2 tbsp brandy
1 egg
1 tsp golden caster sugar
2 tsp custard powder
350ml/12fl oz semi-skimmed milk
½ vanilla pod, split
zest 1 small lemon, pared off in strips
    with a veg peeler
4 tbsp half-fat crème fraîche
25g/1oz butter, softened
4 medium slices good white bread
    (such as a small white farmhouse
    loaf), crusts left on
1 tbsp apricot conserve
¼ tsp icing sugar, for dusting

1 Mix together the apricots, raisins and brandy and leave to soak.
2 Beat the egg, sugar and custard powder in a bowl. Warm the milk until boiling, then gradually whisk into the egg mixture. Add the vanilla pod and lemon zest. Cool for 30 minutes. Whisk the crème fraîche into the milk then strain this through a sieve. Grease an ovenproof dish, about 20 x 25cm, with ¼ teaspoon of the butter.
3 Butter the bread with the remaining butter. Spread over the conserve. Cut each slice into four triangles, then lay half, jam-side up, in the dish. Scatter over half the soaked fruit, then repeat, finishing with any unsoaked brandy. Pour over half the custard over and soak for 15 minutes. Heat oven to 180°C/160°C fan/gas 4.
4 Sit the dish in a roasting tin. Pour the remaining custard over the bread, then half-fill the tin with hot water. Bake for 20 minutes, then raise the heat to 190°C/170°C fan/gas 5. Bake for 5 minutes more until the top is crisp and golden. Dust with icing sugar to serve.

PER SERVING 312 kcals, protein 10g, carbs 41g, fat 12g, sat fat 6g, fibre 2g, sugar 20g, salt 0.83g

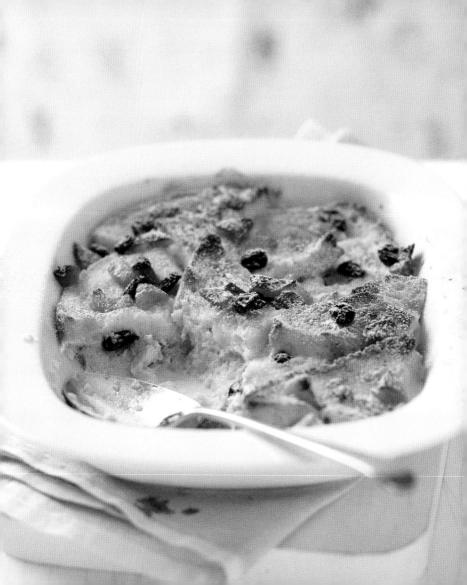

Instant frozen-berry yogurt

Craving something sweet after dinner? Keep a bag of mixed berries in your freezer and this easy pudding is only ever minutes away.

70 KCALS

TAKES 2 MINUTES • SERVES 4

250g/9oz frozen berries,
   plus extra for serving
250g/9oz fat-free Greek yogurt
1 tbsp clear honey or agave syrup

1 Blend the frozen berries, Greek yogurt and honey or agave syrup in a food processor for 20 seconds, until it forms a smooth ice-cream texture.
2 Scoop into four bowls and scatter extra whole berries on top to serve.

PER SERVING 70 kcals, protein 7g, carbs 10g, fat none, sat fat none, fibre 2g, sugar 10g, salt 0.1g

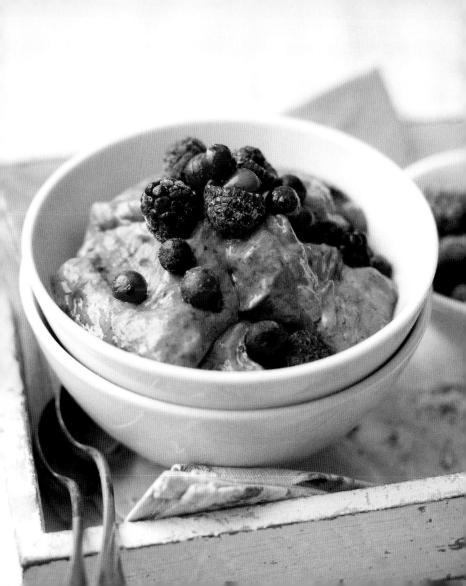

Breakfast bars

These energy-boosting bars will keep for 3 days in an airtight tin – if they hang around that long!

205 KCALS

TAKES 45 MINUTES ● **MAKES 12**

50g/2oz mixed dried fruit (a mixture
of raisins, sultanas and apricots
is nice)
50g/2oz mixed seeds
110g/5oz rolled oats
25g/1oz multi-grain hoop cereal
100g/4oz butter
100g/4oz light muscovado sugar
100g/4oz golden syrup

1 Heat the oven to 160°C/140°C fan/
gas 3. Grease and line a 20cm square tin
with baking parchment. Put the dried
fruit in a mixing bowl. Add the seeds,
oats and cereal and mix well.
2 Put the butter, sugar and golden syrup
in a large pan. Cook gently on the hob,
stirring with the spatula, until the butter
and sugar are melted.
3 Remove from the heat and pour the
dry ingredients into the pan. Mix well
until all the ingredients are coated with
the syrup mix.
4 Fill the baking tin with the mixture. Use
the spatula to press the mix down
evenly. Bake for 20 minutes, then leave
to cool completely before cutting into 12
squares or fingers.

PER BAR 205 kcals, protein 3g, carbs 25g,
fat 10g, sat fat 5g, fibre 2g, sugar 17g, salt 0.2g

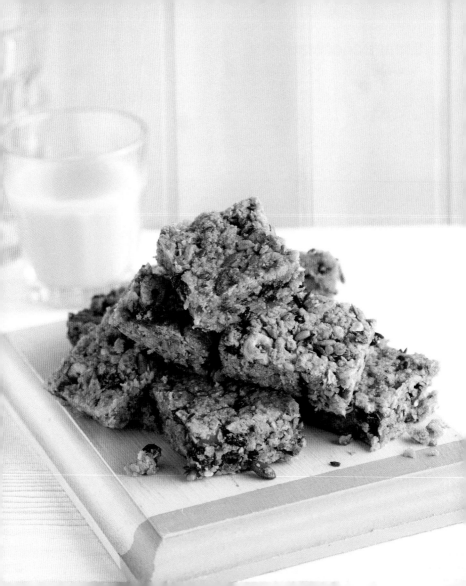

Lighter chocolate tart

Who'd have thought it? A chocolate tart with two-thirds less fat than the classic recipe!

243 KCALS

TAKES 1 HOUR, PLUS CHILLING

● **CUTS INTO 8 SLICES**

FOR THE PASTRY

140g/5oz plain flour, plus extra
　　for dusting
50g/2oz cold butter, cubed
2 tsp cocoa powder
1 tbsp icing sugar
1 tbsp rapeseed oil
1 medium egg yolk

FOR THE FILLING

100g/4oz dark chocolate, 70% cocoa
　　solids, very finely chopped
1 tbsp cocoa powder, plus extra
　　½ tsp for dusting
¾ tsp coffee granules
½ tsp vanilla extract
2 tbsp semi-skimmed milk
2 medium egg whites
2 tbsp dark muscovado sugar
85g/3oz half-fat crème fraîche

1 Rub the flour and butter together until they resemble breadcrumbs. Sift in the cocoa and icing sugar; use a round-bladed knife to stir in the oil, yolk and 2 tablespoons cold water until the dough comes together. Roll out on a lightly floured surface into a circle big enough to fit a 20cm round, shallow, loose-bottomed tart tin with a slight overhang. Prick with a fork. Chill.

2 Heat oven to 190°C/170°C fan/gas 5. Line the pastry with greaseproof paper; fill with baking beans. Bake for 15 minutes. Lift out the beans and paper. Bake for 10 minutes. Trim the excess pastry. Cool.

3 Mix the chocolate, cocoa, coffee, vanilla and milk in a bowl. Sit the bowl over a pan of simmering water, stir, then remove the pan from the heat. Add 2 tbsp of boiling water then leave to cool slightly.

4 Whisk the egg whites until stiff, then whisk in the sugar until glossy. Fold the crème fraîche into the chocolate and very gently add the egg whites, one-third at a time. Remove the pastry from the tin, add the filling. Chill. Dust with cocoa to serve.

PER SLICE 243 kcals, protein 4g, carbs 26g, fat 13g, sat fat 7g, fibre 1.3g, sugar 14g, salt 0.3g

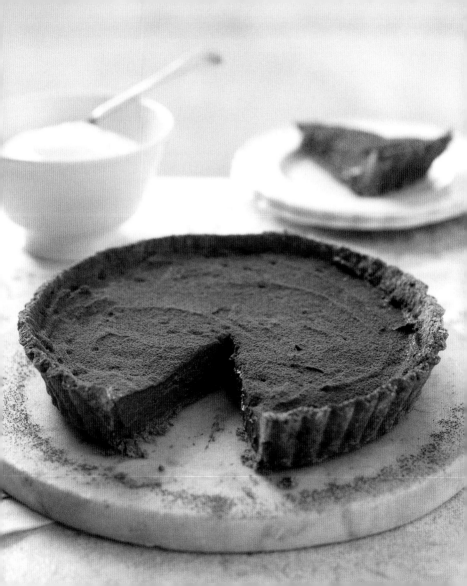

Crunchy custard-baked apples

No need for your diet to be pudding free when these lovely baked apples are this low in fat and calories.

166 KCALS

TAKES 50 MINUTES • SERVES 6

500g carton ready-made custard
(not from the chiller cabinet)
6 Bramley apples, halved through the
middle and core removed
zest and juice 1 orange
1 tsp ground cinnamon
1 tbsp golden caster sugar
6 tbsp crunchy granola with almonds

1 Heat oven to 180°C/160°C fan/gas 4. Pour the custard into a large baking dish. In a large bowl, toss the apples in the orange zest and juice, cinnamon and sugar.
2 Arrange the apples, cut-side up, on top of the custard and drizzle with any extra juice from the bowl. Sprinkle over the granola and bake for 30 minutes, until the apples are soft and piping hot – cover after 20 minutes if the granola is getting dark. Serve with a spoon of low-fat yogurt or a scoop of ice cream, if you like.

PER SERVING 166 kcals, protein 4g, carbs 27g, fat 4g, sat fat none, fibre 3g, sugar 24g, salt 0.1g

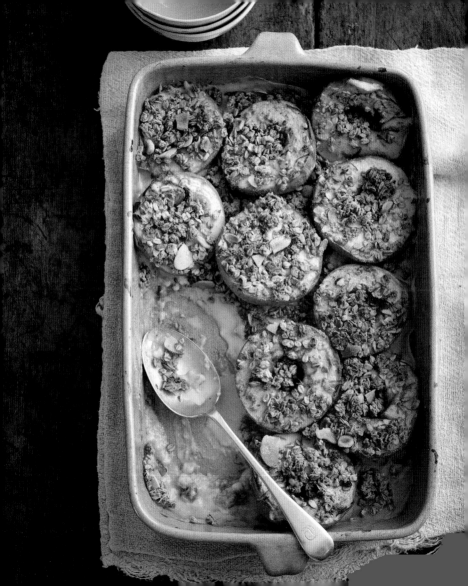

Stem ginger & squash steamed pudding

A sticky steamed pudding is a Sunday-lunch must on a cold day – diet or no diet!

230 KCALS

TAKES 2 HOURS • SERVES 10

butter, for greasing

3 balls stem ginger from a jar,
   finely chopped, plus 4–6 tbsp
   syrup from the jar

3 eggs

200g/7oz golden caster sugar

200g/7oz peeled and finely grated
   butternut squash

zest 1 large lemon

175g/6oz rice flour

50g/2oz ground almonds

2 tsp ground ginger

2 tsp baking powder

1 Lightly butter a 1.5-litre pudding basin. Put one-third of the stem ginger and all the syrup in the bottom.

2 In a bowl, beat the eggs and sugar with an electric whisk until pale and fluffy. Fold in the butternut squash, lemon zest and remaining stem ginger. Fold the remaining dry ingredients into the egg mixture with a large metal spoon until well combined.

3 Fill the basin with the sponge mixture. Cover with a layer of buttered baking parchment and foil, making a pleat in the centre to allow the pudding to rise. Tie on securely with string, then put in a steamer or large pan with an upturned bowl in the bottom. Add boiling water to come halfway up the sides of the basin, cover with a lid and simmer for 1½ hours. Check the water level every now and then, and top up if you need to.

4 To test when the sponge is ready, insert a skewer into the centre. It should come out clean with no trace of raw mixture. Unwrap and serve hot.

PER SERVING 230 kcals, protein 4g, carbs 40g, fat 5g, sat fat 1g, fibre 1g, sugar 26g, salt 0.3g

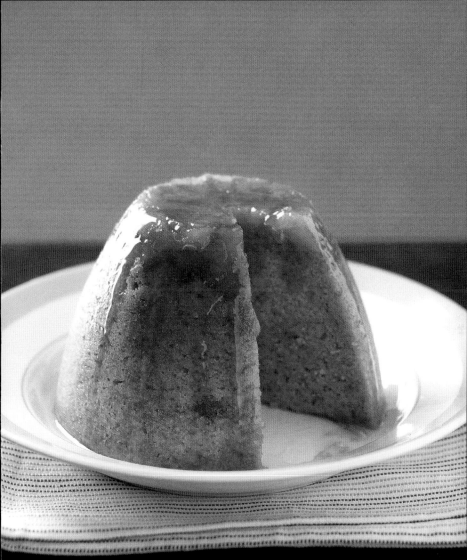

Zesty strawberries with Cointreau

If you're also making this dessert for children, simply splash a little Cointreau over the adult portions when you serve.

69 KCALS

TAKES 5 MINUTES, PLUS
1 HOUR SOAKING • SERVES 4

500g/1lb 2oz strawberries,
    hulled and halved or quartered,
    depending on size
3 tbsp Cointreau
zest 1 orange
4 tbsp icing sugar
mint leaves, roughly torn, to scatter

1 Tip the strawberries into a large bowl. Splash over the Cointreau, add the orange zest and sift in the icing sugar, then give everything a really good mix. Cover, then leave for 1 hour or more for the juices to become syrupy and the strawberries to soak up some of the alcohol.

2 To serve, scatter the mint leaves over the strawberries and give them one more good stir, then spoon into four individual glass dishes.

PER SERVING 69 kcals, protein 1g, carbs 10g, fat none, sat fat none, fibre 1g, sugar 10g, salt 0.02g

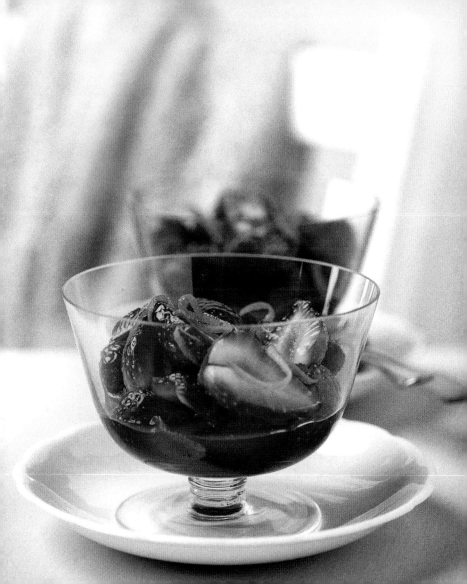

Carrot, courgette & orange cakes

Top decorated cakes with baking parchment, then wrap well in cling film or foil. Freeze for up to a month, then unwrap and defrost, on a serving plate.

273 KCALS

TAKES 45 MINUTES • MAKES TWO 20CM CAKES, EACH CUTS INTO 8 SLICES

250g/9oz butter, softened, plus extra for greasing

200g/7oz caster sugar

3 eggs

250g/9oz self-raising flour

1 tsp bicarbonate of soda

zest 2 oranges

1 tsp ground mixed spice

100g/4oz carrot, grated

100g/4oz courgette, grated

FOR THE ICING

zest 1 orange, plus 2–3 tbsp juice

140g/5oz icing sugar

1 Heat oven to 180°C/160°C fan/gas 4. Grease and line the bases of two 20cm round cake tins with baking parchment. Beat the butter, sugar, eggs, flour, bicarb, orange zest and mixed spice together, then stir in the carrot and courgette. Divide the mixture between the tins and bake for 20–25 minutes or until a skewer inserted into the centre comes out clean. Cool.

2 To make the topping, mix enough of the orange juice with the icing sugar to give a thick but drizzly icing. Drizzle over the cakes, then scatter with the zest and leave to set.

PER SLICE 273 kcals, protein 3g, carbs 35g, fat 14g, sat fat 9g, fibre 1g, sugar 23g, salt 0.54g

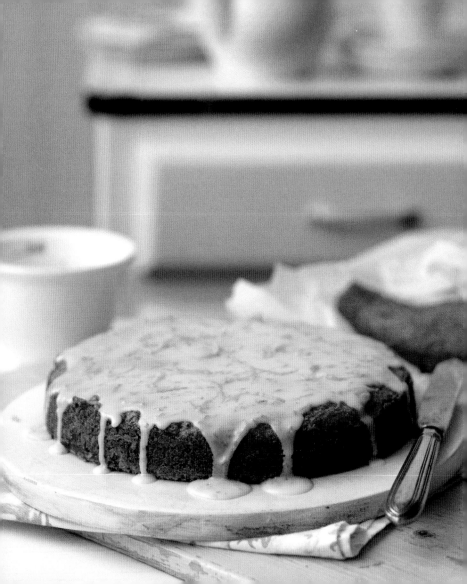

Low-fat cherry cheesecake

Light, luscious and completely make-ahead: perfect for your next dinner party.

342 KCALS

TAKES 1½ HOURS,
PLUS OVERNIGHT CHILLING
● **CUTS INTO 8 SLICES**

25g/1oz butter, melted
140g/5oz amaretti biscuits, crushed
3 sheets leaf gelatine
zest and juice of 1 orange
2 x 250g tubs quark
250g tub ricotta
2 tsp vanilla extract
100g/4oz icing sugar

FOR THE TOPPING
400g/14oz fresh cherries, stoned
5 tbsp cherry jam
1 tbsp cornflour

1 Line the sides of a 20cm round loose-bottomed cake tin with baking parchment. Stir the butter into two-thirds of the biscuit crumbs and press over the base of the tin. Soak the gelatine in a bowl of cold water for 5–10 minutes.
2 Warm the orange juice in a small pan until almost boiling. Squeeze the gelatine of excess water, then dissolve in the juice.
3 Beat the orange zest, quark, ricotta, vanilla and icing sugar with an electric whisk until smooth. With the beaters still running, add the juice mixture. Pour over the biscuit base. Smooth the top. Cover and chill overnight.
4 To make the topping, put the cherries and 100ml/3½fl oz water in a pan. Cook, covered, for 15 minutes. Mash one-third of the cherries to give you a chunky compote. Return to the pan with the jam, cornflour and 2 tablespoons water. Cook until thickened – add a splash more water if needed. Cool.
5 Remove the cheesecake from the tin. Scatter over the remaining biscuit crumbs and some cherry sauce, and serve.

PER SLICE 342 kcals, protein 18g, carbs 47g, fat 9g, sat fat 5g, fibre 1g, sugar 42g, salt 0.3g

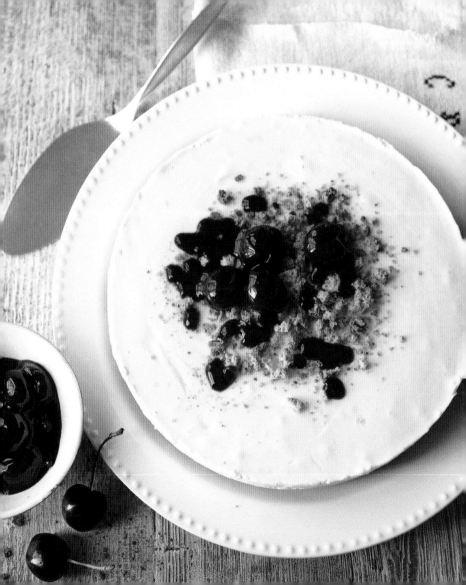

Blueberry & lemon pancakes

For pudding, add a scoop of low-fat frozen yogurt and extra berries to these, or for brunch dollop on some fat-free natural yogurt and a drizzle of agave syrup.

69 KCALS

TAKES 30 MINUTES ● MAKES 14

200g/7oz plain flour
1 tsp cream of tartar
½ tsp bicarbonate of soda
1 tsp golden syrup
75g/2½oz blueberries
zest 1 lemon
200ml/7fl oz milk
1 egg
knob of butter, for cooking

1 Put the flour, cream of tartar and bicarbonate of soda in a bowl and mix well with a fork. Drop the golden syrup into the dry ingredients along with the blueberries and lemon zest.

2 Pour the milk into a measuring jug and beat in the egg. Add most of the milk mixture and mix well. Keep adding more of the milk mix until you get a smooth, thick pouring batter.

3 Heat a frying pan and brush the base with a little butter. Then spoon in the batter, a tablespoon at a time, in heaps. Bubbles will appear on top as the pancakes cook – turn them at this stage. Cook until brown on the second side, then keep warm on a plate, covered with foil. Repeat until all the mixture is used up.

PER PANCAKE 69 kcals, protein 2g, carbs 12g, fat 1g, sat fat 1g, fibre 1g, sugar 2g, salt 0.1g

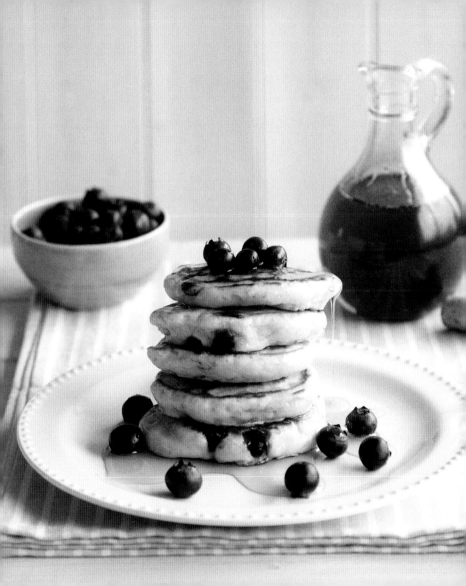

Low-fat tiramisu

A classic Italian dessert reinvented.

220 KCALS

TAKES 45 MINUTES, PLUS COOLING AND OVERNIGHT CHILLING
- **SERVES 8**

250ml/9fl oz strong hot coffee,
   preferably freshly ground
1 tbsp golden caster sugar
4 tbsp Marsala
18 sponge fingers, preferably Savoiardi

FOR THE FILLING

1 tbsp each golden caster sugar and
   cornflour
150ml/¼ pint semi-skimmed milk
1 medium egg, separated
½ vanilla pod, split lengthways
85g/3oz half-fat crème fraîche
1 tbsp Marsala
140g/5oz light mascarpone
100g/4oz light soft cheese
½ tsp cocoa powder, to dust
few raspberries, to decorate

1 Stir the coffee, sugar and Marsala together in a shallow dish. Set aside.
2 Blend the sugar, cornflour and 1 tablespoon of the milk to a paste in a medium pan. Beat in the yolk, then the remaining milk. Transfer to a pan, add the vanilla and stir over a low heat for 8–10 minutes without boiling. Remove from the heat; stir in the crème fraîche and Marsala. Cover with cling film. Cool.
3 To assemble, line a 900g/2lb loaf tin with cling film. Beat together the mascarpone and soft cheese, then stir into the rest of the filling. Whisk the egg white to stiff peaks then fold this in.
4 Briefly dip one of the sponge fingers in the coffee mixture. Lay lengthways in the the tin. Do the same with 5 more, so they cover the bottom of the tin. Spread over half of the filling, then repeat with 6 more biscuits and the remaining filling. Dip and lay the remaining sponge fingers on top. Cover with cling film and chill overnight.
5 Turn out and peel off the cling film. Dust with cocoa and scatter with raspberries.

PER SERVING 220 kcals, protein 6g, carbs 26g, fat 10g, sat fat 6g, fibre 0.3g, sugar 17g, salt 0.25g

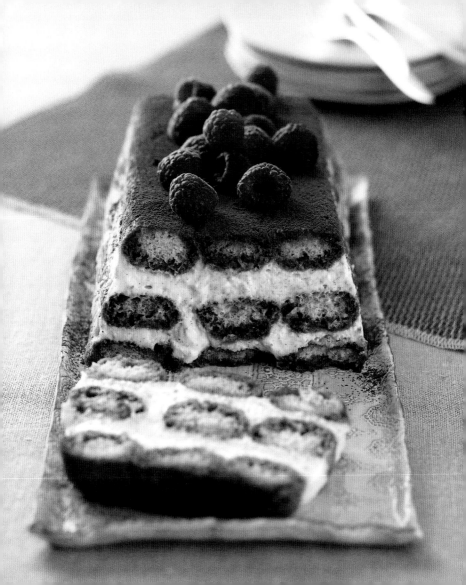

Sticky cinnamon figs

A simple but stylish pudding, ready in just 10 minutes that uses only five ingredients.

162 KCALS

TAKES 10 MINUTES • SERVES 4

8 ripe figs
large knob of butter
4 tbsp clear honey
handful shelled pistachio
   nuts or almonds
1 tsp ground cinnamon
   or mixed spice

1 Heat the grill to medium-high. Cut a deep cross in the top of each fig then ease the top apart like a flower. Sit the figs in a baking dish and drop a small piece of the butter into the centre of each fruit. Drizzle the honey over the figs, then sprinkle with the nuts and spice.

2 Grill for 5 minutes until the figs are softened and the honey and butter make a sticky sauce in the bottom of the dish. Serve warm, with dollops of low-fat crème fraîche or yogurt, if you like.

PER SERVING 162 kcals, protein 3g, carbs 23g, fat 7g, sat fat 2g, fibre 2g, sugar 11.5g, salt 0.06g

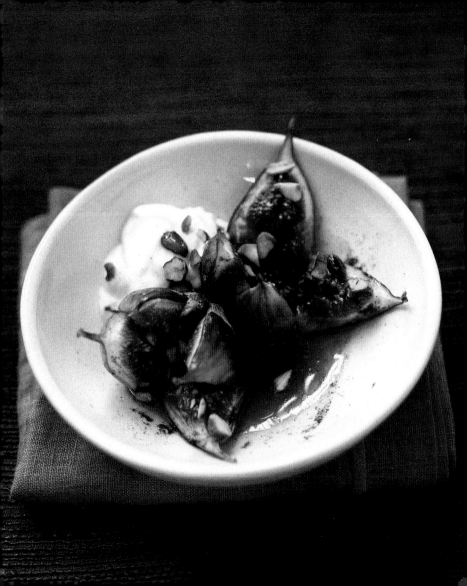

Sticky malt loaves

There's something very satisfying about a cup of tea with a slice of lightly buttered malt loaf – this simple homemade version makes two loaves and improves on keeping.

140 KCALS

TAKES 1 HOUR 5 MINUTES
● **MAKES 2, EACH CUTS**
INTO 10 SLICES

sunflower oil, for greasing
150ml/¼ pint hot black tea
175g/6oz malt extract, plus extra
  for glazing
85g/3oz dark muscovado sugar
300g/10oz mixed dried fruit
2 eggs, beaten
250g/9oz plain flour
1 tsp baking powder
½ tsp bicarbonate of soda

1 Heat oven to 150°C/130°C fan/gas 2. Line the base and ends of two greased 450g/1lb non-stick loaf tins with strips of baking parchment.
2 Pour the hot tea into a mixing bowl with the malt, sugar and dried fruit. Stir well, then add the eggs.
3 Tip in the flour, then quickly stir in the baking powder and bicarbonate of soda and pour into the loaf tins. Bake for 50 minutes until firm and well risen. While still warm, brush with a little more malt to glaze and leave to cool.
4 Remove from the tins. If you can bear not to eat them straight away, the loaves get stickier after wrapping in foil and keeping for 2–5 days, or freeze for up to 2 months well wrapped. Serve sliced and buttered, if you like.

PER SLICE 140 kcals, protein 3g, carbs 31g, fat 1g, sat fat none, fibre 1g, sugar 22g, salt 0.17g

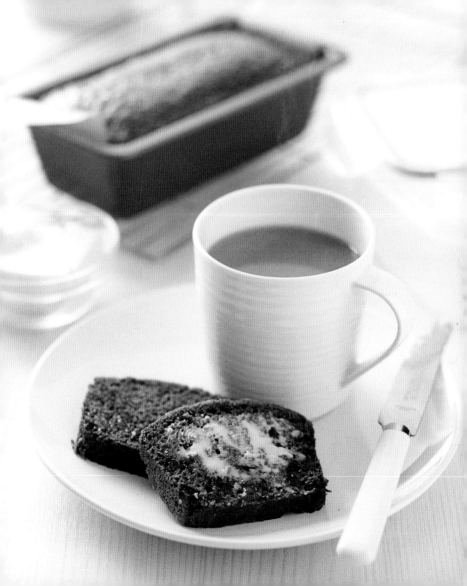

Index

Also available from BBC Books and *Good Food*

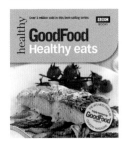

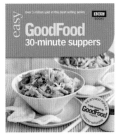

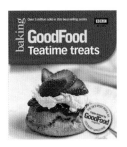

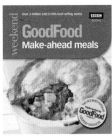

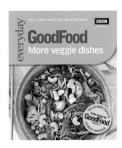

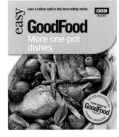

Baking
Cakes & Bakes
Chocolate Treats
Cupcakes & Small Bakes
Easy Baking Recipes
Fruity Puds
Tempting Desserts

Easy
Budget Dishes
Cheap Eats
Easy Student Dinners
Easy Weeknight Suppers
One-pot Dishes
Simple Suppers
Speedy Suppers
Slow Cooker Favourites

Everyday
Best-ever Chicken Recipes
Best-ever Curries
Fish & Seafood Dishes
Gluten-free Recipes
Healthy Family Food
Hot & Spicy Dishes
Italian Feasts
Low-carb Cooking
Meals for Two
Mediterranean Dishes
Pasta & Noodle Dishes
Picnics & Packed Lunches
Recipes for Kids
Stir-fries & Quick Fixes
Storecupboard Suppers

Healthy
Low-fat Feasts
More Low-fat Feasts
Seasonal Salads
Superhealthy Suppers
Veggie Dishes

Weekend
Barbecues and Grills
Christmas Dishes
Delicious Gifts
Dinner-party Dishes
Slow-cooking Recipes
Soups & Sides

Subscribe for £10.50! *

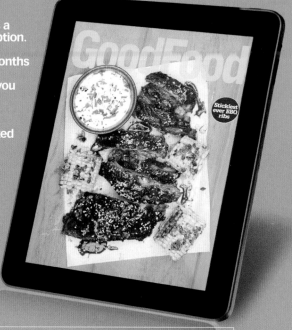

Good Food is now available on iPad as a digital-only subscription.

- Subscribe for 6 months and pay just £1.75 per issue, saving you £7.44 on a 6-issue subscription**.

- Each issue is packed with brand-new recipes, including everyday and seasonal meals. Plus get access to the great interactive features of the app – save and email shopping lists, and watch tutorial videos.

 To get your subscription, and for full terms and conditions, visit *buysubscriptions.com* and click on 'Digital Titles'.